Emergency Nursing Care

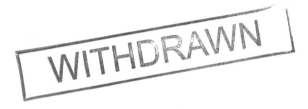

Emergency Nursing Care
Principles and Practice

Edited by
Gary Jones
Ruth Endacott
Robert Crouch

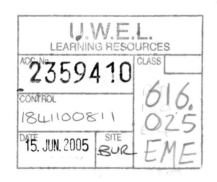

© 2003

Greenwich Medical Media Limited
137 Euston Road
London
NW1 2AA

870 Market Street, Ste 720
San Francisco, CA 94102

ISBN 1 841 100 811

First published 2003

Typeset by Charon Tec Pvt. Ltd, Chennai, India

Printed in the UK by Ashford Colour Press

Distributed by Plymbridge Distributors Ltd and
in the USA by JAMCO Distribution

Visit our website at **www.greenwich-medical.co.uk**

Contents

Contributors

Gary Jones
Fellow Florence Nightingale Foundation
Emergency Nurse Consultant
Lecturer and Expert Witness
UK

Ruth Endacott
Professor of Clinical Nursing
La Trobe University
Bendigo, Australia
Honorary Professor of Clinical Nursing
Institute of Health Studies
University of Plymouth
Plymouth

Robert Crouch
Consultant Nurse
Emergency Department
Southampton General Hospital
Senior Lecturer, School of Nursing and Midwifery
University of Southampton
Southampton

Elizabeth Whelan
Assistant Director of Nursing
Emergency Department
Mater Misercordiae Hospital
Dublin

Maureen O'Reilly
Clinical Nurse Specialist, Emergency Department
Saint Barnabas Medical Center
New Jersey
USA

Mike Heywood
Charge Nurse Emergency Medicine and Lecturer
University of Portsmouth
Portsmouth

Suzanne Knight
Senior Sister
Southampton General Hospital
Southampton

Preface

Emergency care is a broad specialty; emergency nurses have an increasing part to play in its delivery wherever it occurs. Emergency nurses, no matter where they work, require a depth and breadth of knowledge and skill to care for patients with undifferentiated and undiagnosed problems. Many, over the years, have suggested that we are 'Jacks or Jills of all trades and masters of none' – when you start to explore the scope and complexity of emergency nursing it is clear that we are 'masters of emergency care'. The authors desire to explore this complexity and make explicit the knowledge required to practice effectively, was one of the key drivers behind our decision to write this text.

The textbook is based on the main areas of clinical practice identified through the development of the RCN Faculty of Emergency Nursing. The text will be useful to those nurses who use the integrated career and competency framework for professional development. The scope of the book includes frameworks for practice; care of the child and adolescent; adult and older person; minor injury and illness care; mental health; major trauma management; major disasters and incidents.

The text is written, as far as possible, incorporating the best available evidence. Where this is lacking we have used the best-accepted practice. The principles of emergency care are universal; the text is written to reflect this, drawing from international contributors and literature. The book provides background information and quick reference information to assist the practitioner in practice.

We believe that the text has something for everyone, whether new to the specialty or there at its' inception. Everyday presents new challenges; we hope that this text will provide a means to help you meet some of them.

RC, RE, GJ – September, 2002

1 The nature of emergency nursing

Ruth Endacott

Recent policy documents have highlighted the central role of the nurse in the provision of emergency care; this text aims to furnish emergency nurses with a sound underpinning for their diverse role. The wider context for this role is explored in this chapter by defining emergency nursing and articulating the values underpinning its provision. Legal and ethical aspects of practice are explored, together with concepts of teamwork.

DEFINING EMERGENCY NURSING

Emergency care is often ill defined, for example, through the use of terms such as "casualty" or through the grouping of services or courses as "critical care". This has led to misplaced professional and public perceptions of the role of those working in Emergency Departments (Scholes et al 2000). A recent definition of emergency nursing is provided in Figure 1.1.

This definition highlights the following features of contemporary emergency nursing and the wider delivery of health care:

- the patient at the centre,
- the nurse responding to the patient's presentation of their illness,
- the independent and inter-dependent nature of the nursing role,
- the breadth and depth of knowledge and skills required by the emergency nurse.

These principles underpin the approach taken within this text, highlighting areas of knowledge and skill with which the emergency nurse needs to be familiar and practised in order to fulfil the role. The textbook uses groups of patients as the focus for chapter content,

The provision of immediate nursing care to people who have defined their problem(s) as an emergency or where nursing intervention may prevent an emergency arising.

The emergency nurse:
1 accepts without prior warning any person requiring health care with undifferentiated and undiagnosed problems originating from social, psychological, physical, spiritual or cultural factors;
2 leads, initiates and co-ordinates patient care.

- -

Components of the role include:
- rapid patient assessment and assimilation of information often beyond the presenting problem;
- allocation of priorities for care;
- intervention based on the assessment;
- on-going evaluation;
- discharge or referral to other sources of care undertaken independently by the nurse within guidelines.

(RCN 1994a; Endacott et al 1999)

Figure 1.1 Definition of emergency nursing

allowing the reader to explore, for example, specific issues relating to the emergency care of older people.

VALUES UNDERPINNING EMERGENCY NURSING

The way in which emergency care services are designed and delivered reflects underlying values at both local and national level. A review of publications, policy and educational documents suggested that emergency nursing reflects the following key values (Endacott et al 1999) about

- nursing,
- the environment,

- the individual,
- health.

Nursing

Emergency nursing embraces art, science, ethics and use of self. It is more than the response to a set of patient observations, or a series of actions determined by a protocol (for example, Advanced Life Support). In responding to a situation presented by the patient as an emergency, the nurse uses a range of technical, intuitive and personal knowledge in deciding how to best manage the patient.

Environment

Emergency nursing is undertaken in a range of settings and influenced by a wide-ranging socio-political context. The emergency nurse has to be aware of, for example, changes in the provision of primary care, with the development of primary care trusts. Similarly, emergency nursing is defined as the interface between primary and secondary care (Royal College of Nursing, RCN 1994a; Crouch et al 1997), requiring liaison with a range of in-hospital and community services in order to ensure the patient is discharged or transferred to the right environment.

The individual

Emergency nursing emphasizes the individuality of both the patient and the staff; review of journal content emphasizes the value placed on patient's accounts of their experiences in informing nursing practice. Emergency nurses also tailor their patient assessment and management according to the patient's position on a range of continua, for example, their stage of development; age; pre-existing health problems.

Health

Emergency nursing embraces the following beliefs about health:

1 the need to restore health, and return the patient to homeostasis, where possible and facilitate coping for chronic health problems;
2 the need to respond to, and accept, the patient's perception of an emergency;
3 the importance of recognising and responding to local population needs.

The manner in which emergency nursing addresses these four aspects is drawn through in the individual chapters of this text. The overall approach is structured around the different patient groups and the Components of Life nursing model described in Chapter 2.

THE CHANGING POLICY CONTEXT OF EMERGENCY CARE

In the UK, the location of emergency care has changed in focus over the years, with the rapid expansion of nurse-led services such as minor injuries units (Audit Commission 1996) and NHS Direct. This policy shift is also reflected in a more flexible approach to workforce planning, with the suggestion of developing an Emergency Care Practitioner, able to work in the hospital or community setting (JRCALC 1999). This practitioner may come from a range of professional backgrounds, for example, nursing or paramedical training. This emphasizes the need for inter-professional working and inter-professional education, but also provides a driver for the articulation of the unique nursing contribution to emergency care.

There have also been changes in the nursing role in recent years, for example the development of nurse practitioner roles and nurse-led triage. Central to both of these roles is the nurse's key role in patient assessment.

This was emphasized in Sbaih's (1997) ethnographic research study exploring how nurses "become" emergency nurses. However, Sbaih also highlighted the problems arising from the nurses need to safely assess patients but also meet government targets for Patient's Charter. This work also highlighted how the initial patient assessment has the potential to affect the work of the entire department. The central importance of patient assessment in the emergency nurse role is highlighted in this textbook, with coloured textboxes emphasizing key aspects of assessment related to individual patient groups or conditions.

The diversity of patients entering the Emergency Department has been recognized in the past two decades, with a more structured approach to the management of specific patients, for example, the management of children and elderly patients in the Emergency Department; the development of protocols for trauma management; the management of patients presenting with mental health problems. Gender and cultural diversity have also been given greater prominence in approaches to patient assessment and management. The nursing role is central in all these policy developments and has informed the structure of this text.

Shifts in policy thinking are also seen in health department campaigns to encourage patients to seek help from professionals other than emergency care practitioners, for example, pharmacists. This reflects concerns with the heavy workload of Emergency Departments and pre-hospital emergency services. It has also been highlighted through initiatives such as the trolley-waits surveys conducted by the RCN (1994b; 1996), and consumer bodies such as the Community Health Councils. From another angle, there have been numerous studies exploring the "appropriateness" of attendance at Emergency Departments (Jeffery 1979; Sbaih 1993; Walsh 1995) and the reactions of nurses and other professionals to those whose "emergencies" are perceived as non-urgent (Lewis and Bradbury 1982; Byrne and Heyman 1997).

There has also been a move to a culture where the "work" of emergency care is perceived as patient needs that have to be met. Who meets those needs and where they are met is increasingly left to local health services to determine. For example, in some health authorities, all minor injuries will be managed outside of Emergency Departments, whereas in other settings this remains part of the Emergency Department role. This policy shift is reflected in this text, with the emphasis on the care required by the patient (*emergency care*) rather than the location (*the Emergency Department*).

LEGAL DIMENSIONS OF CARE

The legal context, in which emergency nurses work, is defined and debated in detail elsewhere. However, it is crucial for the nurse to understand the central tenet of accountability for his/her actions, and the indirect accountability for actions delegated to others by the nurse.

Four main arenas of accountability in law are of particular relevance to nurses:

■ The Public = Criminal liability
■ The Patient = Civil liability
■ The Profession = Professional liability
■ The Employer = Employment liability.

Whilst all areas of law are seeking to protect the common goal of individual rights and, specifically for

health care, protecting the public, the potential for conflict between these areas can be seen where an incident is viewed by an employer as a breach of contract but not seen by the NMC as unprofessional conduct. In this scenario, a nurse could be sacked by his employer but not removed from the professional register.

Accountability has been usefully defined as follows:

The ability to demonstrate the necessary competency, skill and knowledge to take charge of a case, knowing the limits of one's ability to carry out that charge and having the confidence gained from experience and up-to-date knowledge to decide what has to be done and to do it (Kitson 1993).

This emphasizes the need for nurses to also have the authority and autonomy to make decisions about the management of the patient (for example, requesting radiographs). Nurse-led services such as minor injuries units are often in the forefront of these debates.

FORMULA FOR ESTABLISHING NEGLIGENCE

In discussing the legal context of emergency care, it is helpful to focus on the nurse's accountability to ensure that care given is not negligent. In addressing this issue, a court of law would ask the following three questions:

1 Was a duty of care owed by the defendant (trust) to the plaintiff (patient/relative)?
2 Was the standard of care broken?
3 Did the breach in the standard of care cause the plaintiff harm?

The acceptable standard of care is determined by both national and local policies (see Figure 1.2).

In the UK, the extent to which individual trusts meet the acceptable standard of care is reflected in the level of indemnity they are awarded against claims of negligence. This is administered by the NHS litigation authority through the Clinical Negligence Scheme for Trusts (CNST) and is usually embraced within the Trust's Clinical Governance strategy.

The move towards a culture of "no blame" should mean that any errors or adverse incidents are more likely to be reported. Moreover, Lord Woolf proposed that doctors, and other health care professionals, should be obliged, as part of their ethical code, to report

The nature of emergency nursing

National standards
NMC standards
DoH guidance
RCN publications
Resuscitation Council guidelines
Marsden manual of clinical policies and procedures
Health and safety at work legislation

Local standards
Prescribing protocols
Admission/discharge protocols
Infection control policies

Figure 1.2 National and local standards underpinning emergency care

to the patient any act or omission in their care that may have caused injury, and that doctors (and other health care professionals) who fail to comply should be subject to disciplinary action (Lord Woolf 2000).

The overall means of achieving an "open" culture could be summarized as

- identifying not *who* went wrong but *what* went wrong,
- talking through the incident rather than instigating an investigation,
- treating the incident as a training point rather than a disciplinary matter,
- learning lessons and changing systems as appropriate.

ETHICAL ASPECTS OF EMERGENCY NURSING

The centrality of ethics in emergency nursing is almost inevitable given the nature of the situations that present themselves on a daily basis. Tschudin (1992) helpfully defines ethics as follows:

Ethics are involved at the boundary of what is acceptable and what is not (yet) acceptable.

Whenever ethical issues are discussed in emergency nursing, they are likely to centre around one or more of the five key ethical principles (see Figure 1.3). These issues may be discussed on the *macro* level, when decisions are made about the emergency care service, or at the *micro* level in the Emergency Department when facing a situation of ethical difficulty with an individual patient.

- *Respect for the individual*
  The need to ensure confidentiality and privacy.
- *Respect for the autonomy of the individual*
  The need to ensure appropriate consent is given by the patient or relative.
- *Beneficence/non-malfeasance*
  The need to ensure that decisions regarding treatment for the individual patient are designed to be of benefit to the patient, not merely to avoid harm.
- *Honesty*
  That individual patients and families are given honest information regarding progress and prognosis. This ethical principle also relates to Lord Woolf's assertion that health care professionals admit their mistakes to the patient (see above).
- *Justice*
  Equity of access rather than postcode services.

Figure 1.3 Five key ethical principles (after Beauchamp and Childress 1989)

Of these issues, the matter of informed consent is one which troubles many health care professionals. Following an audit of informed consent in one NHS Trust, Campbell and Gladstone (2000) used the following principles to educate clinicians:

1. description of the procedure should be in words which the patient can understand, with no abbreviations,
2. the person signing the consent form should be a competent clinician – one who could potentially undertake the procedure,
3. clinicians should use any opportunity to record discussions about informed consent in the case notes,
4. clinicians can add relevant risk information to the consent form.

There is no legal requirement for the patients' signature on the consent form to be witnessed. However, it is essential that patients and their families are given sufficient explanation of the procedures for which they are consenting. In some departments where this activity is likely to be undertaken by a diverse number of staff, it may be helpful to define, for each procedure, what constitutes "explanation of the procedure". An overview of the law on consent has been published by the Department of Health (DH 2001) and is reproduced in Figure 1.4.

When do health professionals need consent from patients?

1 Before you examine, treat or care for competent adult patients you must obtain their consent.

2 Adults are always assumed to be competent unless demonstrated otherwise. If you have doubts about their competence, the question to ask is: "can this patient understand and weigh up the information needed to make this decision?" Unexpected decisions do not prove the patient is incompetent, but may indicate a need for further information or explanation.

3 Patients may be competent to make some health care decisions, even if they are not competent to make others.

4 Giving and obtaining consent is usually a process, not a one-off event. Patients can change their minds and withdraw consent at any time. If there is any doubt, you should always check that the patient still consents to your caring for or treating them.

Can children consent for themselves?

5 Before examining, treating or caring for a child, you must also seek consent. Young people aged 16 or 17 are presumed to have the competence to give consent for themselves. Younger children who understand fully what is involved in the proposed procedure can also give consent (although their parents will ideally be involved). In other cases, someone with parental responsibility must give consent on the child's behalf, unless they cannot be reached in an emergency. If a competent child consents to treatment, a parent *cannot* over-ride that consent. Legally, a parent can consent if a competent child refuses, but it is likely that taking such a serious step will be rare.

Who is the right person to seek consent?

6 It is always best for the person actually treating the patient to seek the patient's consent. However, you may seek consent on behalf of colleagues if you are capable of performing the procedure in question, or if you have been specifically trained to seek consent for that procedure.

What information should be provided?

7 Patients need sufficient information before they can decide whether to give their consent: for example, information about the benefits and risks of the proposed treatment, and alternative treatments. If the patient is not offered as much information as they reasonably need to make their decision, and in a form they can understand, their consent may not be valid.

Is the patient's consent voluntary?

8 Consent must be given voluntarily: not under any form of duress or undue influence from health professionals, family or friends.

Does it matter *how* the patient gives consent?

9 No: consent can be written, oral or non-verbal. A signature on a consent form does not itself prove that the consent is valid – the point of the form is to record the patient's decision, and also increasingly, the discussions that have taken place. Your trust or organization may have a policy setting out when you need to obtain written consent.

Refusal of treatment

10 Competent adult patients are entitled to refuse treatment, even where it would clearly benefit their health. The only exception to this rule is when the treatment is for a mental disorder and the patient is detained under the 1983 Mental Health Act. A competent pregnant woman may refuse any treatment, even if this would be detrimental to the fetus.

Adults who are not competent to give consent

11 No one can give consent on behalf of an incompetent adult. However, you may still treat such a patient if the treatment would be in their best interests. "Best interests" go wider than best medical interests, to include factors such as the wishes and beliefs of the patient when competent, their general well-being and their spiritual and religious welfare. People close to the patient may be able to give you information on some of these factors. Where the patient has never been competent, relatives, carers and friends may be best placed to advise on the patient's needs and preferences.

12 If an incompetent patient has clearly indicated in the past, while competent, that they would refuse treatment in certain circumstances (an "advance refusal"), and those circumstances arise, you must abide by that refusal.

Figure 1.4 Twelve key points on consent: the law in England (DH 2001)

Article 1	The Convention
Article 2	Right to Life
Article 3	Prohibition of Torture
Article 4	Prohibition of Slavery and Forced Labour
Article 5	Right to Liberty and Security
Article 6	Right to a Fair Trial
Article 7	No Punishment without Law
Article 8	Right to Respect for Private and Family Life
Article 9	Freedom of Thought
Article 10	Freedom of Expression
Article 11	Freedom of Assembly and Association
Article 12	Right to Marry and Found a Family
Article 14	Prohibition of Discrimination
Article 16	Restrictions on Political Activity of Aliens
Article 17	Prohibition of Abuse of Rights
Article 18	Limitations on Use of Restrictions on Rights

Figure 1.5 Articles of the Human Rights Act (1998)

These ethical issues are explored further in individual chapters relating to the management of different patient groups.

The importance of these considerations in everyday relationships is highlighted through the publication of the Human Rights Act (1998), derived from the European Convention on Human Rights. The act contains 18 articles, identified in Figure 1.5.

A helpful analysis of the implications of the act for practitioners in the NHS has been provided by the NHS Litigation Authority (NHSLA 2000) and is reproduced in Figure 1.6. Wilkinson and Caulfield (2000) provide a more detailed outline of the act as it applies to nursing practice. The full text of the act can be found at www.homeoffice.gov.uk/hract

This flowchart provides a useful framework for decisions regarding new and existing policies and procedures for emergency nursing in your setting. You need to be able to demonstrate that you have considered the convention rights and taken appropriate action to ensure that practice is compatible with the act.

One area of practice that has received much publicity in recent years, and is highlighted in several articles of the act, is the issue of racism. Following the McPherson report on institutionalized racism within the Metropolitan police the RCN discussed this issue at its congress. The question was raised regarding racism within the health care services and the RCN.

Since that debate the RCN has promoted diversity awareness through a number of key activities. Staff and activists have had specific training and RCN offices hold a range of events celebrating diversity and supporting a number of network groups. A diversity resource guide has been developed which supports activists in assessing employers' policies and progress in managing diversity and equality.

The RCN has also pioneered an innovative Connect Project, which examines strategies for cultural diversity networks, communication and learning. The project builds alliances with city councils, health authorities, trusts and community organizations.

TEAM CONCEPTS

Emergency nursing is not practised in isolation; the success of interventions is likely to be dependent on the contributions of many practitioners, from the Paramedic and Fire and Rescue Personnel in the pre-hospital setting to the consultant anaesthetist and radiographer. In order to work effectively in a team, key features are required. These are presented in Figure 1.7 (p. 8).

Teamwork can be promoted and "practised" through the use of simulation where poor teamwork and communication have been demonstrated, practising team roles using simulation has been demonstrated to improve teamwork (Santora et al 1996). However, teamwork is also a key to the success of "everyday" situations. The diverse nature of emergency nursing, with patients from across the entire age range, disease range and cultural range, emphasizes the need for the nursing team to develop complementary roles, as the goal of being competent in all those dimensions of care is largely unattainable for the individual nurse. Hence there is a need to recognize, value and develop the individual contributions of team members. This process starts with the preceptorship of new staff and builds through mentoring, clinical supervision and appraisal processes.

The key to effective emergency nursing care is the development of a team of nurses, with appropriate knowledge and skills, who work with other professionals to respond to emergency situations. The

Ruth Endacott

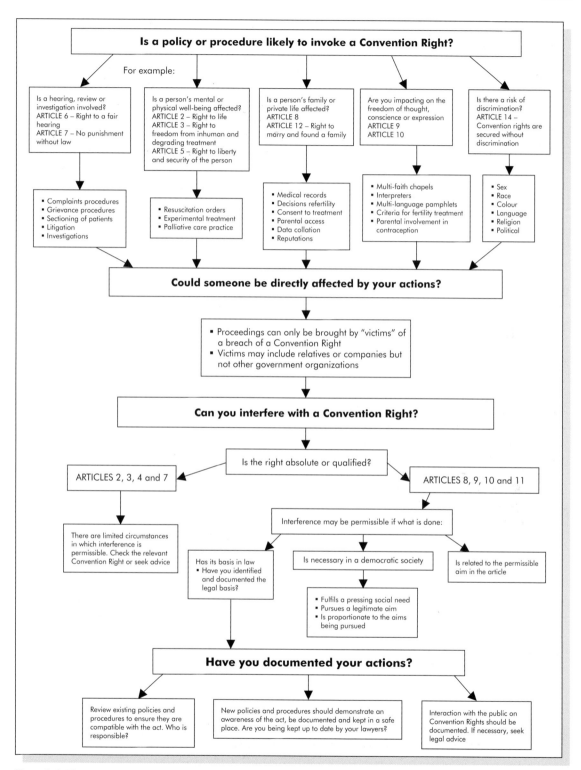

Figure 1.6 The Human Rights Act 1998 – Checklist for the NHS (reproduced with permission, NHSLA Review issue 19–2000)

> ■ Effective verbal communication
> ■ Effective written communication
> ■ Enabling and encouraging supervision
> ■ Culture that encourages team members to seek help
> ■ Collaboration
> ■ Common goals
> ■ Valuing the contribution of individual members
> ■ Matching team roles to ability
> ■ Team structure (consistency; directional and supportive leadership)
>
> (Adapted from: Vincent et al 1998)

Figure 1.7   Key elements of teamwork

remaining chapters in this text provide a foundation for that process.

References

Audit Commission (1996) *By accident or design? Improving A&E services in England and Wales.* London: HMSO.

Beauchamp and Childress (1989) *Biomedical ethics,* 3rd ed. New York: Oxford University Press.

Byrne G, Heyman R (1997) Understanding nurses: communication with patients in accident and emergency departments using a symbolic interactionist perspective. *J Adv Nurs* 26(1): 93–100.

Campbell B, Gladstone J (2000) Informed consent: how to improve conformity and compliance. *NHSLA Rev* 18: 16–17.

Crouch R, Haverty S, Westcott J, Dale J (1997) Primary care in the A&E department: meeting the challenge: a workshop series for A&E nurses. *Nurs Edu Today* 17(5): 481–486.

DH (2001) *Twelve key points on consent: the law in England.* London: HMSO.

Endacott R, Crouch R, Edwards B et al (1999) Towards a faculty of emergency nursing. *Emergen Nurs* 7(5): 10–16.

Jeffery R (1979) Normal rubbish: deviant patients in casualty departments. *Sociol Health Ill* 1(1): 90–107.

JRCALC, Joint Royal Colleges Ambulance Liaison Committee (1999) *The practitioner in emergency care.* London: JRCALC.

Kitson A (1993) Accountable for quality. *Nurs Stand* (Euroquan suppl) 8(1): 4–6.

Lewis B, Bradbury Y (1982) The role of the nursing profession in hospital accident and emergency departments. *J Adv Nurs* 7(3): 211–221.

Lord Woolf (2000) *Access to justice.* London: HMSO.

NHS Litigation Authority (2000) *NHSLA Rev* 19.

RCN (1994a) *Accident and emergency: challenging the boundaries.* London: RCN.

RCN (1994b) *Waiting for a bed.* London: RCN.

RCN (1996) *Still waiting for a bed.* London: RCN.

Santora TA, Trooskin SZ, Blank CA, Clarke JR, Schino MA (1996) Video assessment of trauma response: adherence to ATLS protocols. *Am J Emergen Med* 14(6): 564–569.

Sbaih L (1993) Accident and emergency work: a review of some of the literature. *J Adv Nurs* 18: 957–962.

Sbaih L (1997) Becoming an A&E nurse. *Accid Emergen Nurs* 5(4): 193–197.

Scholes J, Endacott R, Chellel A (2000) To prime or to consolidate experience? A review of ENB 199 A&E courses. *Accid Emergen Nurs* 8: 34–41.

Tschudin V (1992) *Ethics in nursing: the caring relationship,* 2nd ed. Oxford Butterworth-Hienemann.

Vincent CA, Adams S, Stanhope N (1998) A framework for the analysis of risk and safety in medicines. *Br Med J* 316: 1154–1157.

Walsh M (1995) The health belief model and use of accident and emergency services by the general public. *J Adv Nurs* 22: 694–699.

Wilkinson R, Caulfield H (2000) *The Human Rights Act: a practical guide for nurses.* London: Whurr.

2 | Care of the emergency patient – frameworks for nursing assessment and management

Gary Jones

This chapter provides the reader with an insight into various models and frameworks used within emergency care and focuses specifically on the Components of Life framework. Throughout the chapter the use of the Components of Life framework is linked with clinical conditions that commonly present to the emergency care setting showing how a structured approach to nursing care can be achieved. More details regarding individual "conditions" can be found in the subsequent chapters.

INTRODUCTION

While most patients require emergency care for physical problems (conditions) many others will require care stemming from a psychological or social source. In addition the emergency nurse provides care to relatives and friends of the patient. Spiritual and cultural factors are also important when caring for an individual.

Provision of good emergency nursing care results from the nurse working in a structured and logical way. The very nature of emergency nursing requires the use of a model or framework that underpins the assessment, planning, intervention and evaluation process.

Emergency nursing frameworks are seen in such tools as the SOAPE format (Blythin 1988), triage (Mackway-Jones 1996) and trauma care (TNCC 2000).

These frameworks do not encompass major theorist philosophies but rather provide a structure on which to build the patient assessment, intervention and evaluation. No one tool is used in isolation, each one compliments the other.

THE TRIAGE FRAMEWORKS

Triage (allocation of a priority for care) has been used in the emergency care setting for many years. Until the mid-1990s there was no agreed national standards or priority categories and many Emergency Departments developed in-house systems often based on previous work (Blythin 1988; Jones 1988). In 1996 the Royal College of Nursing Emergency Department Association with the British Association for Emergency Department Medicine agreed a UK national triage scale based on a five-point framework. This framework places the patient into one of five priority categories (Crouch and Marrow 1996; Marrow 1998). The Manchester Triage System (Mackway-Jones 1996) (Figure 2.1) has been adopted by a large number of emergency care settings and this methodology is now the most commonly used. The Manchester system links comfortably with the agreed national triage scale and uses flow charts based on presenting conditions in adults and children such as chest pain, headache and abdominal pain. The tool also uses discriminators such as pain, which automatically places the patient into a specific priority category.

Frameworks for nursing assessment and management

Immediate resuscitation (red)
- Patients in need of immediate treatment for the preservation of life
- No delay
- Patient usually met by a team on arrival

Very urgent (orange)
- Seriously ill or injured patients whose lives are not in immediate danger
- Should be seen within 10 min of arrival

Urgent (yellow)
- Patients with serious problems, but apparently in a stable condition
- Should be seen within 60 min of arrival

Standard (green)
- Standard Emergency Department cases without immediate danger or distress
- Aim to see within 120 min

Non-urgent (blue)
- Patients whose conditions are not true accidents or emergencies
- Should not have to wait for more than 240 min

Figure 2.1 Manchester Triage System

While triage is about setting priorities for care, in its day to day use it encompasses a number of goals including:

Goals of triage (Jones 1990)
- Early patient assessment
- Priority rating
- Assignment to correct area of care and infection control
- Control of patient flow
- Initiation of diagnostic measures
- Initiation of emergency care
- Patient education.

TRAUMA CARE FRAMEWORKS

In trauma care a simple framework based on the alphabet has been used very successfully over the last 10–15 years. The most recent update of the framework (TNCC 2000) uses an A–I mnemonic (Figure 2.2). It is not intended to encompass the whole person but simply provides the essential structure to the primary and secondary survey. This is explored in greater detail in Chapter 7.

NURSING CARE MODELS AND FRAMEWORKS

Throughout the last 20 years nursing has seen the development of theories and nursing models. A nursing model is based on a philosophy (belief and values) about humans being the recipients of nursing and includes achievable goals and the knowledge and skills on which nursing practice is based. Names such as Henderson, Roper, Orem, Rogers and Roy are just some that reflect the number of nursing theories and models available. The majority of models were developed from the theorist conceiving an idea, expounding and developing it into a model, then putting it into practice. While some of these models were (and still are) implemented in wards and departments many other models and frameworks have been developed from analysing practice and developing a usable tool from what actually exists.

A practice-based approach to the development of nursing models was given credibility by Wright (1986) and has been used by many since. Jones (1990) used this approach to develop the Components of Life model. This model was developed from practice within an Emergency Department and was introduced into emergency nursing in 1986 after an extensive piece of work at the authors own Emergency Department in England. The model in various formats is now used in a number of Emergency Departments throughout the UK. It has also been referenced in work from Australia, and the USA. The model has been validated by a number of emergency nurses and lecturers within emergency care. Through independent work it has been shown that the model provides a definition of the four metaparadigms as described by Fawcett (1989).

The original Components of Life model was based on seven components that are all reflected within emergency nursing practice. A new Components of Life framework retains the components in a slightly

Primary assessment

A = **Airway** – assess for a clear or obstructed airway; if obstructed, clear the airway.

B = **Breathing** – assess for breathing and any life-threatening chest injury; treat as necessary.

C = **Circulation** – assess for circulation and any life-threatening wounds; treat as necessary.

D = **Disability (disorders of consciousness)** – assess the level of consciousness; treat as necessary.

Secondary assessment

E = **Exposing the injury/environmental control** – appropriate to the environment and reminds you to maintain the casualty's body temperature.

F = **Full set of vital signs/five interventions** – cardiac monitor, pulse oximeter, urinary catheter, gastric tube, laboratory studies, facilitate family presence.

G = **Give comfort measures** – verbal reassurance, touch.

H = **Head to toe assessment** – start at the head and inspect/feel every part of the body.

I = **Inspect the back** – assess for any injury to the back.

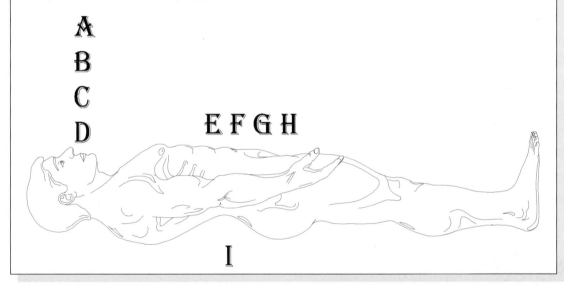

Figure 2.2 The A–I mnemonic

revised format (Figures 2.3a (p. 12) and 2.3b (p. 13)). Linked with four universal goals (Figure 2.4 (p. 14)), the components provided a framework on which nursing care is developed and nursing documentation maintained. Given a numerical scoring, the components are used to determine the dependency of the patient for nursing care as well as acting as a tool to support the management of the emergency care setting.

THE COMPONENTS OF LIFE FRAMEWORK

Following a number of departments using the original model and work within a number of Emergency

Departments on developing both nursing records and dependency measurement tools, the original model has been revised. The revised framework links more readily with the Jones Dependency Tool (JDT), which itself originates from the model but through research (Crouch, Williams and Jones 2001) has been refined.

USING THE FRAMEWORK

Dependent on the environment in which emergency nursing care is provided will determine the patient's first contact with the emergency nursing service. Nurses providing emergency care via a telephone advice service will treat the initial telephone contact

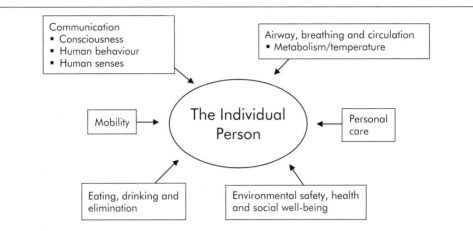

Communication
Humans are social beings who through communication and relationship with others achieve much of their quality of life. Partnership is developed through communication and information is shared. Human behaviour communicates much of the person's attitude, moods, religious beliefs, sexual identity and emotions. The physiological senses are also important in the establishment of good communications.

Airway, breathing and circulation
Oxygen is vital to life. To ensure normal tissue activity, a clear airway, normal respiratory function and adequate circulation is essential.

Mobility
The ability to move enables the individual to engage in work and play. It provides the individual with independence and social well-being.

Personal care
The ability to maintain personal care allows the individual to retain good hygiene and reduce the risk of ill-health through infection.

Eating, drinking and elimination
Health is maintained by the adequate intake of food and water. Through normal digestive and metabolic activities the body is able to function normally and eliminate waste.

Environmental safety, health and social well-being
Individuals require a safe environment and the recognition of self-care to maintain health. Depending on the individual's work, lifestyle and attitude, the degree of risk will vary.

Individuals have a desire to remain in good health. Economic as well as social circumstances have a bearing on the individuals ability to maintain health. A balance often has to be achieved between the wish to remain healthy and social activities that can put health at risk.

Social well-being is very individual but for many will include good health, mobility, the ability to communicate and interrelate with others, rest, a stable living environment and financial well-being.

Figure 2.3(a) The Components of Life framework

with the patient as the arrival. In the Emergency Department or minor injury/walk in unit the physical presence of the individual will be considered as the arrival.

Irrespective of the arrival mode, the nurse must establish communication with the patient and begin to establish a partnership arrangement. It can be seen that even at this very early stage a component from the nursing framework (communication) is being used and an attempt made to achieve one of the universal goals (achieving a partnership).

As the assessment progresses so other components will be used to create a total picture of the patient's problems. Concurrently the nurse will begin to

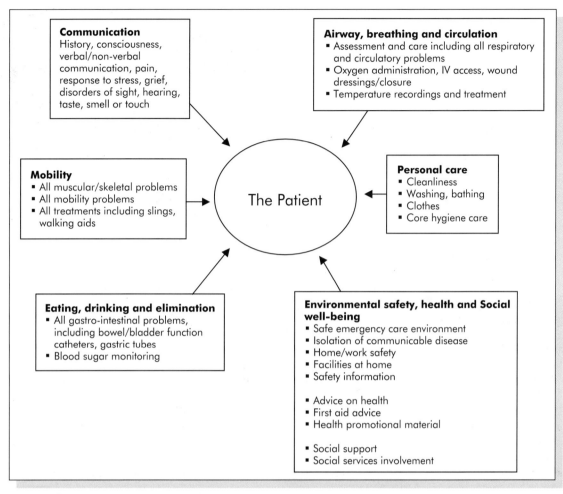

Communication
History, consciousness, verbal/non-verbal communication, pain, response to stress, grief, disorders of sight, hearing, taste, smell or touch

Airway, breathing and circulation
- Assessment and care including all respiratory and circulatory problems
- Oxygen administration, IV access, wound dressings/closure
- Temperature recordings and treatment

Mobility
- All muscular/skeletal problems
- All mobility problems
- All treatments including slings, walking aids

The Patient

Personal care
- Cleanliness
- Washing, bathing
- Clothes
- Core hygiene care

Eating, drinking and elimination
- All gastro-intestinal problems, including bowel/bladder function catheters, gastric tubes
- Blood sugar monitoring

Environmental safety, health and Social well-being
- Safe emergency care environment
- Isolation of communicable disease
- Home/work safety
- Facilities at home
- Safety information

- Advice on health
- First aid advice
- Health promotional material

- Social support
- Social services involvement

Figure 2.3(b) Using the Components of Life framework

identify how easy (or difficult) it is going to be to achieve the other universal goals. A plan of action will be established which will include individual goals linked to the four universal goals and intervention carried out. By using the six key components of the framework it is easy for the nurse to identify all interventions under the key headings, establish individual goals and with the universal and individual goals, evaluation of the process of care is relatively easy.

- Establish individual goals linked to the four universal goals
- Provide planned care based on the assessment
- Evaluate care – have the goals been achieved?

COMMUNICATION

Communication and the establishment of a partnership between the nurse and patient may not be a simple process. Communication in itself is a very complex activity yet it is essential if the nurse is to understand why the patient requires emergency care (history) and for ongoing intervention. Numerous factors will influence communication and partnership including the

The structured approach
- Patient arrives
- Assessment using the six components
- Allocate a triage and dependency score

Frameworks for nursing assessment and management

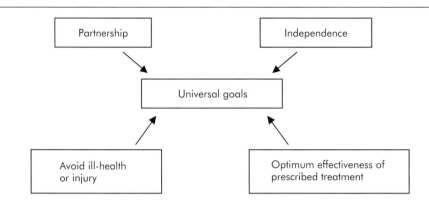

To establish a partnership with the patient/relatives
Partnership is established through communication. Both parties need to be committed to the establishment of a partnership. Attitude, prejudice, age, social background, drugs, alcohol are just some of the many influences that challenge the establishment of a partnership.

To achieve a level of independence in the patient appropriate to the illness or injury
Although independence is desirable, in many patients full independence may not be achievable in the short term. Some patients will be totally dependent on the nurse while others will have varying degrees of dependency. This universal goal must be linked with specific goals that are set in partnership with the individual and the overall dependency for nursing care.

To enable the individual to avoid ill-health or injury through self-care, health education and environmental safety
The emergency nurse must strive to assist the patient to maintain health and prevent injury. Health education and safety advice must be an integral part of emergency nursing.

To ensure the optimum effectiveness of nursing and medically prescribed treatment is obtained
It is essential that patients understand the rational behind the treatments prescribed and their part in effecting recovery. Correct care of wound dressings and medication taken at the correct dose and time are just two examples of the patient's part in the recovery process.

Figure 2.4 The four universal goals

patient's level of consciousness, human behaviour and human senses.

Consciousness

The patient's conscious level will greatly influence the amount of communication that is possible. Consciousness can be measured in fairly simple or very complex ways. The most simple method is to use the AVPU tool (see Figure 2.5). This tool provides the nurse with an initial awareness of the patient's consciousness ranging from fully alert with eyes open and an apparent awareness of what is happening (Alert) through to no response to pain (Unresponsive). Response to Verbal stimulation suggests the patient continues to drift into a state of sleeplessness but is stimulated by sound. Response to Pain includes

- Approach the patient
- Identify if the patient is looking towards you and appears to respond. If so the patient can be described as
  ALERT   A
- If the patient responds to voice and then closes the eyes until verbally stimulated again, then the patient is described as responding to
  VERBAL STIMULI   V
- If the patient only responds when pain is inflicted (pinching the back of the hand or pressing the nail bed) then this response is responding to **PAIN STIMULI**   P
- Finally if no response is achieved, the patient is **UNRESPONSIVE** (unconscious)   U

Figure 2.5 Assessment of consciousness using the AVPU tool

Eyes open	Spontaneously	4
	To speech	3
	To pain	2
	None	1
Best verbal response	Orientated	5
	Confused	4
	Inappropriate words	3
	Incomprehensible sounds	2
	None	1
Best motor response	Obey commands	6
	Localize pain	5
	Withdraws from pain (normal flexion)	4
	Abnormal flexion to pain	3
	Extension to Pain	2
	None	1

Figure 2.6 The Glasgow Coma Score

verbal response or limb movement. While this tool does not provide a great deal of information it is an acceptable method during the initial (primary) assessment of the patient.

Ongoing use of AVPU

A response moving to alertness is a good sign. However, patients moving in the opposite direction are deteriorating.

A more detailed means of determining the patient's consciousness uses the Glasgow Coma Scale (Score) (Figure 2.6). The Glasgow Coma Score (GCS) provides an objective, standardized and easily interpreted tool for neurological assessment (Dawson and Sanders 2000). It removes the ambiguity around such words as "semiconscious" that can clearly mean different things to different people. The GCS is made up of three activities – eye response, verbal response and motor response. Each section ranges from full response to no response. Unconsciousness is an imprecise term usually meaning an unaware patient with whom verbal communication is not possible; unresponsive is thus a better description (Moulton and Yates 1999).

The GCS ranges from 15 (fully conscious) to 3 (no response); however, this tool is never used in isolation. Incorporated within what is often described as the GCS chart is the simultaneous recording of blood pressure, pulse, respiration, temperature, pupil reaction and limb movements. Recording all of these vital

signs together means a reasonable accurate picture of the patient's condition can be obtained.

Changes in the neurological score are very significant and will often indicate signs of deterioration well before any other parameter changes.

If the patient is unresponsive then the assessment/ intervention/evaluation will move immediately to the airway/breathing/circulation. If, however, the patient's consciousness enables the nurse to conduct a history, the intervention and evaluation will come later.

Human behaviour

Human behaviour is another important aspect of establishing communication and partnership. It is the product of life transitions and affects the way we respond within society. Communication and partnership may be enhanced or destroyed by the human behaviour of both the patient and the nurse. Attitude, religious beliefs, moods, sexual identity and emotion are just a few of the human behavioural traits that will influence the way communication and the partnership is developed. Other factors include culture, whether the person is assertive, passive or aggressive and if the use of drugs and alcohol are involved. Non-verbal communication is helpful during the assessment of a patient but this is one major area of communication that is not available to the nurse providing a telephone consultation. In this situation verbal communication and understanding between both parties are essential.

Human senses

Communication is also established through our senses – sight, hearing, taste, smell and touch. Touch is particularly important and can provide the therapeutic relationship to achieve optimum support of physical and emotional needs. Pain is a major communication factor that can influence the quality of patient assessment. If a patient is in pain and the pain is not relieved quickly, the partnership can easily break down and the detailed history that is required will not be forthcoming. Pain is one of the key discriminators in the Manchester Triage scoring methodology (Mackway-Jones 1996).

Frameworks for nursing assessment and management

History

Fundamental to identifying the patient's problem(s) is the history. Various factors have already been identified as having an influence on how well or how poorly the history will be obtained. Taking a history is like playing detective – searching for clues, collecting information without bias yet staying on track to solve the puzzle (Clark 1999).

People who attend the Emergency Department come with a range of very different problems. While the history from relatives/friends or passers by is often very helpful, the ability to obtain a history from the patient is important and can often be crucial. Research by Marsden (2000) shows that when a nurse practitioner is able to obtain a history and question a patient directly (either by telephone or face to face) a correct provisional diagnosis can be made more accurately than when the information is provided by other health care personnel. Marsden also identified (as have others in previous work) that the skill of

the nurse in obtaining the history by asking the right questions and having a sound knowledge base is essential.

In many physical conditions the agent that has caused the problem and the mechanism in which the agent has entered or has come in contact with the patient can be identified. The mechanism of injury or illness is therefore key to an accurate diagnosis (Figure 2.7).

Illness as opposed to trauma (a wound or injury caused by external force or violence (Blackwell's Dictionary of Nursing 1994) can either be acute (sudden onset), chronic (slow onset) or an acute on chronic condition. With infection, the common agent that causes the illness can be bacteria or virus. The way in which the infection enters the body (the mechanism) will often determine where the infection occurs. In some cases the infection can be isolated to a specific area of the body, in others the infection may spread throughout all body systems.

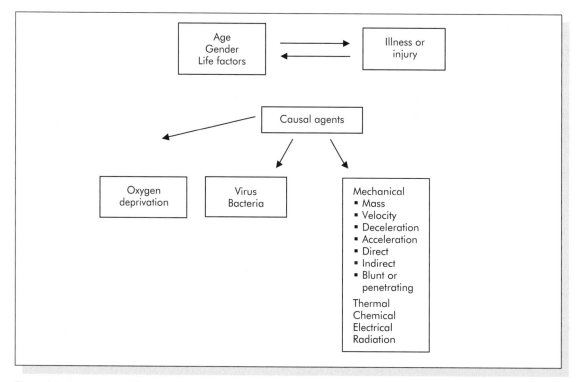

Figure 2.7 Mechanism of illness and injury

Irrespective of the agent, be it infective, neoplastic or degenerative, it will in some way or other injure the structure of the human body, this injury will not only be seen in an anatomical or physiological way but it will also effect the individuals social and emotional status.

Injury due to trauma is the result of an external energy force that has come in contact with the body. The most common mechanism of injury (how the energy reaches the body) is from a mechanical source such as a car, fall, knife, gun, etc. Other sources include heat, chemicals, electricity and radiation (TNCC 2000).

The mechanism of injury due to trauma is particularly important because it is often the key factor in the management of the trauma patient (see Chapter 7).

Many conditions will cause a sudden reduction in the body's oxygen levels. While some of these will be trauma related, others will be as a direct result of illness (the body's inability to utilize the oxygen) or the inability of the body to receive oxygen from the air (drowning, smoke filled room). Whatever the mechanism that has caused the reduction, the end result will be injury to the body tissues.

By talking (communicating) with the patient/relative, asking relevant questions and listening to the answers a picture of the current reason for requesting emergency care can be established and a partnership developed. The types of questions will depend on the chief complaint, however general history required from most patients will include:

General history
- Chief complaint
- Mechanism of injury or illness
- Past medical history (if relevant)
- Any medication being taken
- Immunization status (especially tetanus).

To use a literary quote:
— *their names are What and Where and When and How and Why and Who (Kipling).*

Ongoing communication

The continuation of communication and partnership throughout the intervention and evaluation stages of the patient's time in the emergency care setting is essential. One common complaint from patients is the absence of communication from staff, especially throughout any waiting periods (Jones 1995). While nurses may feel uncomfortable or even threatened by a large volume of patients in a waiting room, a lack of communication will only heighten the possible breakdown of the partnership that is so essential for ongoing care of the individual.

AIRWAY, BREATHING AND CIRCULATION

A clear airway, normal breathing and good circulation are all essential for life. While the accepted practice is to assess and intervene for each sub-component in turn (A then B then C), all three are inextricably linked and within the team concept are supported simultaneously (Figure 2.8).

Airway

Reflecting on the use of specific goals to support the universal goals within the Components of Life framework, the establishment of a clear airway can demonstrate how these two link. One of the universal goals is to achieve a level of independence in the patient appropriate to his/her condition. If a patient is unresponsive and unable to manage his/her own airway then the nurse will identify a specific goal – to establish a clear airway. The airway once clear will enable the patient to breath and therefore a level of patient independence will have been established.

Breathing and circulation

Breathing and circulation involves looking, listening and feeling. Wounds to the chest may affect both; skin colour reflects the adequacy or inadequacy of breathing as well as the circulation. If required, intervention involves supporting both breathing and circulation. While circulation may require a number of interventions including wound closure and the administration of intravenous (IV) fluids, the administration of high percentage oxygen will benefit both.

Oxygen is essential to life; it was first isolated separately by Priestly and by Scheele in 1774 (Clynes et al 1973). It is the most abundant element in the

Assessment

■ **Look**
- In the airway – for blood, vomit, foreign bodies, oedema, tongue obstruction
- At the chest – for movement, rate and depth of respirations, use of accessory muscles, symmetrical breathing pattern or asymmetrical breathing patterns
- At the skin – for integrity, wounds, bruising, texture, colour

■ **Listen**
- For noise in the airway – gurgling, snoring, wheeze
- Silent or noisy breathing – sucking chest wound

■ **Feel**
- For air on your cheek
- Major pulses, rate, volume and rhythm

Look, Listen and Feel for 10 seconds

Intervention

If necessary, establish a clear airway by correct position – chin lift or jaw thrust with or without head tilt (do not use head tilt if cervical spine injury is suspected)

Any fluid in the airway must be removed by the use of position and/or suction

The airway can be maintained with the use of the oro-pharyngeal or nasal pharyngeal airways or if necessary the laryngeal mask or endotracheal intubation

Provide
- ■ Oxygen or ventilation as required
- ■ Chest compression if necessary
- ■ Pressure dressings to wounds
- ■ Appropriate positioning of the patient depending on the problem

Evaluation

Has the intervention achieved the objectives? If not reassessment is required and further intervention established.

Figure 2.8 Airway, breathing and circulation – the first few minutes

earth's crust and occurs in the air to an extent of 21–23% of the total gases. Therapeutic oxygen is manufactured and is 99.5% pure. Foss (1990) indicates that oxygen administration has two effects. The first is the increased diffusion of oxygen across the alveoli membrane. This is attributed to raised alveoli oxygen tension that therapy produces. The second effect is due to 2 ml of oxygen being dissolved in every 100 ml of blood.

Although a medical practitioner prescribes oxygen, most if not all Emergency Departments should have standing orders/patient group directions that allow nursing staff to administer oxygen when the patient's condition requires. The decision to administer oxygen and the percentage required will depend on the patient's history, signs and symptoms, and condition. In most departments three types of mask will be required. A fixed flow rate mask at 24% or 28%. A variable flow rate mask for the majority of acute conditions and the non-rebreathing mask for the patient

with severe oxygen deficiency, e.g. the multiple injured patient or the acute cardiac/respiratory patient. All acute conditions, e.g. trauma, myocardial infarction and asthma, require high levels of oxygen, e.g. 60–100%.

Circulation can be disrupted by a number of problems (commonly trauma, various heart conditions or other medical ailments). Many of these can result in shock.

Shock

There are numerous definitions of shock. Any definition must focus on the cell, since cellular death is central to all forms of shock (Zoellner-Hunter 1990). Howarth and Evans (1994) describe shock as an abnormality of the circulation leading to inadequate organ perfusion and tissue oxygenation. While there are a number of causes of shock, any condition, physical or psychological, which reduces the heart's ability to pump or reduces venous return, is a potential cause of shock (Richardson 2000).

Common causes of shock are hypovolaemia (reduction in body fluid), cardiac (reduction in the heart's ability to pump at a normal pressure), neurogenic (reduction of normal autonomic responses), septic (infective agent) and anaphylaxis (extreme allergy reaction). All can be seen within emergency nursing and the emergency nurse not only needs to distinguish the type of shock but also needs to be aware of the correct intervention.

The body's response to shock

Irrespective of the cause, a sudden reduction in the blood pressure leads to an inadequate blood supply to all body tissues, which in turn leads to inadequate tissue oxygenation. To overcome this major event the body activates a major response in an attempt to increase the blood pressure and thereby improve organ perfusion and tissue oxygenation. Figure 2.9 shows in a simplified format how the body responds to the sudden drop in blood pressure. While this response is of benefit in the hypovolaemic patient

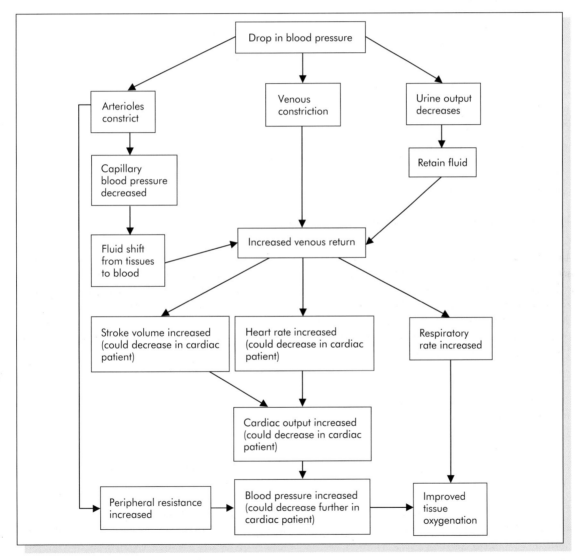

Figure 2.9 The body's response to shock

the same response can cause increased problems to the patient with cardiogenic shock. In anaphylactic shock the body's response may not be achieved without drug assistance.

Assessment

The cause of the shock will often determine the presenting signs and symptoms. However, in the majority of patients many of the signs and symptoms are similar because of the reduced blood pressure and inadequate tissue oxygenation.

Key to a good assessment is the history and identification of any obvious complaints such as trauma, external wounds, chest pain or a known allergy.

Intervention/evaluation

Although specific interventions such as IV fluids and drugs will be determined by the cause of the shock, general principles include:

- Positioning of the patient
- Oxygen administration
- Reassurance
- Maintaining body temperature
- Regular evaluation of vital signs including pulse, respirations, blood pressure, urine output and general mental state.

The management of different types of shock is covered in detail in Chapter 7.

Metabolism and body temperature

Airway, breathing and circulation provide the essentials for normal metabolism. Any disruption of this component will have a direct effect on the metabolism of the body. Metabolic disorders while being complex will normally result in a change in the body temperature. When using the components as a framework for nursing care, temperature changes can be properly identified under this component heading.

MOBILITY

Injury whether due to illness or injury will often affect normal mobility. Mobility is often linked closely to the individual's ability to mix socially and can profoundly affect the individual's physical and psychological stability. As an emergency nurse it is essential to establish what is the patient's normal mobility and how has the present illness or injury affected the mobility. This information will be obtained during the assessment and is an essential part of the history taking.

Dependent on the patient's problem, assessment of the mobility component will either focus on one part of the body, e.g. the arm or a whole body mobility problem. The assessment begins when the patient arrives. The patient limping towards the nurse will often display mobility problems affecting one leg. Arm injuries will often be supported either by the patient holding the arm or with the use of a temporary sling. The patient in a wheelchair or on a stretcher suggests a more significant loss of mobility.

The restrictions that the mobility problem places on the individual will be dependent on the cause and subsequent treatment as well as the patient's overall health and fitness. The universal goal of achieving independence in the patient appropriate to his/ her condition is well illustrated with this component. A young fit person with an ankle injury will be able to maintain far more independence than a person with the same injury who has an underlying chronic condition.

During the assessment the nurse must establish the degree of mobility loss.

If the loss is due to an injury is there any
- deformity?
- joint displacement?
- swelling?
- pain?
- lack of movement/sensation?

Mobility loss can be due to muscular or neurological problems – assess for normal muscle tone, sensory and motor function.

Intervention under this component heading will be determined by the problem and could range from supporting an injured arm in a sling through to frequently turning a patient to prevent pressure sore development.

Again under this component heading we can see how components interlink and also the interlinking with the universal goals. If we take a patient who has been provided with a sling to support an arm injury we can see how good communication and the partnership approach will allow the patient to understand the need to maintain the arm sling. The correct use of the arm sling ensures the optimum effectiveness of the prescribed treatment (another of the universal goals).

PERSONAL CARE

The amount of personal care that the individual requires from the nurse will be determined by the overall condition. Assessment of the personal care component involves a general overview of the clothes and shoes, the hair, hands and face. More detailed assessment involves undressing the patient and inspecting all skin surfaces. The nurse must not become judgmental as dirty clothes; hands and face may simply reflect the type of work an individual undertakes. Dirty underwear can suggest poor personal care and while psychological conditions may cause the patient to neglect personal care, more commonly a reduction in mobility will determine the amount of personal care that can be achieved.

While providing personal care is a core nursing activity, assessing the patient's personal care ability especially as part of discharge planning is essential and should always be carried out by a registered nurse. Apart from the ability of the patient to wash, bath or dress, the nurse must also link this component to others such as eating, drinking and elimination, and environmental safety. It must also be linked with the universal goals – avoiding injury through self-care and achieving independence.

EATING, DRINKING AND ELIMINATION

While adequate fluids and nutrition are essential for life both are normally restricted during emergency care, especially the injured person. Many conditions seen in the emergency care setting can be linked with problems of eating, drinking and elimination. Poor diet results in a vast range of medical conditions and increased weight can be the cause of chronic musculoskeletal problems. When assessing a patient with any abdominal or bowel related problems, or a person suffering from weight loss; any changes in diet,

digestion, swallowing or bowel habits must be identified. Inadequate carbohydrate intake in an insulin dependent person will result in a sudden reduction of glucose and diminished/altered consciousness. Increased blood glucose levels can cause various manifestations and routine check of the blood glucose is essential in all patients with diminished levels of consciousness, infected skin lesions, fits and in children complaining of abdominal pain.

Abnormalities in elimination can range from urinary retention through to various digestive problems. Direct observation of the urine, faeces or vomit is essential. The amount, colour, content and smell often assists in identifying the problem. Routine testing of the urine using an impregnated stick will show up many abnormalities.

ENVIRONMENTAL SAFETY, HEALTH AND SOCIAL WELL-BEING
Environmental safety

Environmental safety can be subdivided into two:

- The person's home and workplace.
- Within the care setting (Emergency Department/ minor injury clinic).

Many injuries seen within the emergency care setting are often the result of a lack of environmental safety in the home, on the road or in the workplace. Eye injuries can occur in the workplace due to the non-use of safety glasses. Head injuries can be due to the lack of safety helmets. The arm injury may be due to a lack of a guard on the machine or the person's own reluctance to use it.

In the home a loose carpet can be the cause of a fall especially in the elderly. The lack of a handrail on the stairs or on the bath can also lead to falls and major limb injuries. People suffering from some medical conditions may be working in environments that are potentially hazardous and children in the home are always at risk due to their natural curiosity.

When nursing any individual we should also be aware of the needs of relatives. The patient may have an elderly relative at home that is at risk, a child may be expecting the mother to arrive at the end of school time and if the mother is not there the child could be at risk. The nurse has a responsibility to ensure other agencies are informed so such risks are reduced, e.g. ringing the school or contacting social services.

When providing nursing care to a patient the nurse can use this opportunity to introduce environmental safety advice. A worker with a corneal foreign body is more likely to appreciate the need for using safety glasses while being treated than being told several months after the injury. The same applies to patients going home especially the elderly. What hazard caused the visit and what can be done to prevent this happening again? Support from occupational therapy and social services may be required.

Within the care setting the nurse has a responsibility to ensure all patients, the nurse and colleagues are safe. Under Health and Safety legislation the employer also has a responsibility. Isolating potentially infectious patients, use of trolley sides and staff training are all ways of ensuring environmental safety is maintained.

Health

Ill health can often be due to a lack of personal health care. While health promotion can be difficult the emergency nurse should not loose the opportunity to promote health whenever possible.

While it is inappropriate to suggest to a patient in the acute stages of a myocardial infarction that smoking may have contributed to the present problem it is appropriate for the nurse to discuss cross infection with a patient suffering from conjunctivitis. It is also very appropriate to discuss health promotion with someone who has just suffered a hypoglycaemic episode due to a lack of breakfast. Explanation as to how first aid measures can contribute to reducing problems in the initial few minutes of an injury is another way of nurses promoting health.

Many nurses contribute to health promotion through the use of visual displays in the waiting rooms and many will also hold specific theme days. These displays and theme days will often link environmental safety and health promotion.

Social well-being

While all the components have an influence over an individual's social well-being, it is important to identify those patients and relatives that may require

support within the community. The universal goal of independence appropriate to the patient's condition can for some, only be achieved with additional support. Early assessment and intervention can help patients and relatives remain within the community.

DEPENDENCY SCORING USING THE JONES DEPENDENCY TOOL

As previously stated, the original Components of Life model and now the updated framework have been used to determine patient dependency. Blackwell's Dictionary of Nursing (1994) defines dependency as a condition of being dependent on someone or something. What the JDT provides is a method of identifying the patient's dependency for nursing care and then links that dependency with a nursing workload.

The tool is in two sections, Section A provides six key component headings with each one having three ratings of dependency ranging from total dependence to total independence (Figure 2.10). On arrival and subsequently throughout the stay in the Emergency Department this section provides the dependency score of the patient. Based on the dependency score a number of actions can be implemented:

1 The nurse allocated to the patient should have the relevant competencies to provide care for the patients' dependency.
2 The dependency rating across the department at any given time can be calculated and actions taken if a threshold level is reached.

Section B reflects the nursing workload that the patient dependency creates and is generated by each of the four dependency scores. Under each dependency heading is a number of nursing interventions – direct and indirect (Figure 2.11, p. 24). These interventions reflect nursing time (direct and indirect). This section can be used to determine nursing numbers and with dependency/competency factors can determine skill mix.

During 2000/2001 the JDT through research project funded by the NHS Executive, was refined and validated in a multi-centre study (Crouch, Williams and Jones 2001). The results provided evidence that the refined JDT is a reliable and valid instrument for

Choose one box (3, 2, 1) from each component (one or more factors in the box is sufficient to receive your allocation). Place each rating in the rating column. Then add the ratings to give a total JDT rating.

Component	3	2	1	Rating
Jones Dependency Tool (JDT)				
Communication	■ Complete impairment due to either loss of one or more senses ■ Pain being at the higher range of the visual analogue scale ■ Unresponsive ■ Language barrier ■ Extensive behavioural problems	■ Impairment or potential for impairment of one or more senses ■ Pain at the mid-range of the visual analogue scale ■ Responding only to verbal/pain stimulation ■ Difficulty due to language barrier ■ Anxious/tearful/distressed	■ Able to communicate through all senses ■ Pain at the lower range of the visual analogue scale ■ Alert ■ No language barrier ■ Co-operative/relaxed	
ABC	■ Cardiac/respiratory arrest (or risk of arrest) ■ Complete impairment of ABC or shock	■ Risk of impairment to airway breathing or circulation ■ Potential for shock due to condition	■ No ABC problems ■ Minor wounds	
Mobility	■ Total immobility	■ Partial mobility loss ■ Patient requires trolley/wheelchair	■ Fully mobile ■ Minor limb problem	
Eating, drinking, elimination and personal care	■ Total loss of bowel/bladder function and/or hyperemesis ■ Total loss of independent self-care	■ Partial loss of bowel/bladder function and/or vomiting ■ Partial loss of independent self-care	■ Normal bowel/bladder control; no vomiting ■ Able to maintain independent self-care	
Environmental safety, health and social needs	■ Demonstrates danger to self or others ■ Appears to require extensive social support	■ Appears unable to fully understand risks ■ Appears to require some social support	■ Shows total ability to fully understand risks ■ Does not appear to require social support	
Triage	■ Red or orange	■ Yellow	■ Green or blue	
			Total JDT rating =	
Dependency score based on total rating score 6–7 Low dependency = 0 8–12 Moderate dependency = 1	13–15 High dependency = 2 16–18 Total dependency = 3		Dependency score	

Figure 2.10 Jones Dependency Tool, Section A (Crown copyright, 2000; with permission)

measuring adult patient dependency in the Emergency Department.

NURSING RECORDS

Recording the nursing assessment, intervention and evaluation is essential. The Nursing and Midwifery Council believe that record keeping is a fundamental part of nursing and that the quality of your record keeping is also a reflection of the standard of your professional practice.

For general day-to-day use the Components of Life framework provides the structured headings under which nursing records can be made. For trauma patients specific records can be designed around the A–I framework.

The design of any nursing record will be determined by a number of factors including the preference

Frameworks for nursing assessment and management

Jones Dependency Tool (JDT)				
Component	Total dependency 3	High dependency 2	Moderate dependency 1	Low dependency 0
Communication	■ Nurse present at all times (one to one) (D/I) ■ Constant attention due to behavioural problems/need for psychological support (D) ■ Constant support/ frequent contact with relatives (I) ■ May require analgesia IM/IV	■ Constant observation (but not requiring one to one) (D/I) ■ Frequent attention due to behavioural problems/need for psychological support (D) ■ Frequent support/ contact of relatives/ friends due to severity/ death of patient (I) ■ May require analgesia IM/IV	■ Nurse available in calling distance (D/I) ■ Reassurance/ psychological support (D) ■ May require relatives to be informed/ explanation (I) ■ May require analgesia IM/IV	■ Nurse available in the department (D/I) ■ Reassurance (D)
ABC	■ Frequent (15 min) vital signs (D) ■ Constant airway/ breathing attention (D) ■ Resuscitation (D) ■ Rapid IV fluids (D) ■ Extensive or time consuming interventions/tests (D/I)	■ Vital signs 1/2–1 hourly (D) ■ Observation/ intervention with airway/breathing (oxygen administration) (D) ■ Frequent IV fluids (D) ■ Require various blood tests (D/I)	■ Vital signs 2–4 hourly (D) ■ IV fluids (D)	■ Vital signs once only (D)
Mobility	■ Frequent pressure area care (D) ■ Constant elimination support (D) ■ Extensive or time consuming interventions/tests (D/I)	■ Pressure area care 1–2 hours (D) ■ Require X-rays/scans (D/I)	■ Pressure area care 4/6 hourly (D)	■ Nil specific
Eating, drinking Elimination and personal care	■ Requires constant attention to care	■ Assistance with bedpans/urinals (D)	■ Assistance with toiletry/commode/ walking to toilet (D)	■ Nil specific
Environmental safety, health and social needs	■ Constant attention due to behavioural problems (D) ■ If discharged, will require complex discharge arrangements involving more than one service provider (I) ■ Admission planning (I) ■ Will require escorting to wards/departments (D) ■ Extensive time consuming health promotion/self-care advice required (D)	■ Frequent attention due to behavioural problems (D) ■ If discharged, will require complex discharge arrangements involving more than one service provider (I) ■ May require admission planning (I) ■ Will require escorting to wards/departments (D) ■ More extensive health promotion/self-care advice required (D)	■ May require some discharge planning linked with one service provider (I) ■ May require admission planning (I) ■ May require escorting to wards/departments (D) ■ Requires some health promotion/self-care guidance (D)	■ Discharge planning is uncomplicated (I) ■ Some health promotion/ self-care may be required (D)

Nursing workload: D, direct care; I, indirect care.

Figure 2.11 Jones Dependency Tool, Section B (Crown copyright, 2000; with permission)

Gary Jones

for the following:

- Stand-alone nursing records or an inter-professional record?
- All nurses to record in the same manner?
- Separate records for minor vs major illness/injury?
- Tick boxes, blank sheets or some of each?
- A record to incorporate all patient data or use add on sheets?
- A record that incorporates observation chart/fluid chart?
- A computer or hand written record?

Other factors to consider include:

- Time creating the records should be as short as possible.
- The records must act as guidance for nurses (education tool and aid memoir).
- What about storage?

All nursing records should contain the patient's biographical details, and a logical process

- History
- Assessment (subjective and objective information)
- Plan and goal setting (can be excluded if intervention immediately follows the assessment and the plan and goal are clearly identified within the assessment/intervention records)
- Intervention
- Evaluation.

Remember the plan and intervention must reflect the assessment. The patient must be involved and the records should demonstrate – a discussion with the patient, patient consent, information given to the patient and any issue regarding confidentiality.

Common errors that are seen in many nursing records must be avoided. Dimond (1995) indicates some common errors in record keeping:

- Times omitted
- Illegible handwriting
- Abbreviations which are ambiguous
- Use of tippex
- No signature

- Lack of information
- Inaccuracies especially dates
- Lack of patient data
- Meaningless phrases, e.g. "nice patient"
- Unprofessional terminology, e.g. "thick as two short planks"
- Opinion mixed with facts
- Subjective and objective information mixed.

Remember any document is a legal document. Missing documents need to be accounted for. Any errors should be scored through so that they can still be read.

CONCLUSION

As previously stated no one emergency care framework can stand in isolation. The early patient assessment, infection control, emergency care and patient education goals that are fundamental to the triage process are all inexplicably linked with the Components of Life framework. Similarly the A–I framework for trauma care has many cross-links with the Components of Life. Using any framework or model provides a structure to your care and allows for good nursing records.

References

Blackwell's Dictionary of Nursing (1994) Oxford: Blackwell.
Blythin P (1988) Triage in the UK. *Nursing* 3(31): 16–20.
Clark C (1999) Taking a history. In: Walsh M, Crumbie A, Reveley S, eds. *Nurse practitioners – clinical skills and professional issues*. Oxford: Butterworth Heinemann.
Clynes S, Williams D, Clarke J (1973) *A new chemistry*. English Universities Press.
Crouch R, Marrow J (1996) Towards a UK triage scale. *Emergen Nurs* 4(3): 4–5.
Crouch R, Williams S, Jones G (2001) *Patient dependency in A&E: validation of the Jones Dependency Tool (JDT)*. Report to Department of Health, England.
Dawson D, Sanders K (2000) In: Dolan B, Holt L, eds. *Accident and emergency – theory into practice*. London: Baillier Tindall.
Diamond B (1995) Legal Aspects of Nursing. Hemel Hempstead: Prentice Hall.
Emergency Nurses Association (2000) *Trauma nursing core course manual*. Emergency Nurses Association, Chicago.
Fawcett J (1989) *Analysis and evaluation of conceptual models of nursing*, 2nd ed. Philadelphia: Davis & Company.
Foss MA (1990) Oxygen therapy. *Profess Nurs* 5(4): 188–190.
Howarth P, Evans R (1994) *Key topics in accident and emergency medicine*. Oxford: Bios publishers.

Jones G (1988) Top priority. *Nurs Stand* 3(7): 28–29.

Jones G (1990) *Accident and emergency nursing – a structured approach*. London: Faber & Faber.

Jones G (1995) Initial Assessment in A&E. Report to the Patient's Charter Unit. Department of Health, Leeds. Summary of Report published in Patients' Charter News issue 21 September 1995 NHS Executive, Leeds.

Mackway-Jones K, ed. (1996) *Emergency triage: Manchester Triage Group*. London: BMJ.

Marrow J (1998) National triage scale exists. *Br Med J* 317: 207 (18 July) letters.

Marsden J (2000) Telephone Triage in an Ophthalmic A&E Department. London: Whurr Publisher.

Moulton C, Yates D (1999) *Emergency medicine*, 2nd ed. Oxford: Blackwell Science.

Richardson M (2000) Physiology of practice. In: Dolan B, Holt L, eds. *Accident and emergency – theory into practice*. London: Baillier Tindall.

Wright S (1986) Building and using a model of nursing. Edward Arnold, London.

Zoellner-Hunter J (1990) In: *Emergency nursing – a physiologic and clinical perspective*. Philadelphia: Saunders.

3 | Emergency care of the child and adolescent

Suzanne Knight and Robert Crouch

Children and adolescents (0–16 years inclusive) make up 25–30% of annual attendee's at Emergency Departments (EDs) (Royal College of Nursing 1998). By the age of five, 44% of all children will have sustained an injury that requires treatment and care in an ED (Muller et al 1992). The arrival of an injured or acutely unwell child into the ED can cause considerable anxiety to staff. To allay these fears, knowledge of the anatomical and physiological differences, response to illness and injury as well as an understanding of how to manage the ill or injured child are required. The ability to assess and treat children and adolescents can be challenging for even the most experienced nurse.

The following chapter aims to highlight the key aspects of knowledge required by emergency nurses in the care of the child and adolescent in the ED. This chapter is not exhaustive but covers a number of the most common presenting illnesses to the ED.

CHILDHOOD DEVELOPMENT

The Children Act 1989 states that a child is someone up to his or her 18th birthday. The term "child" is defined as covering the age range *"from birth to puberty"* (Concise Oxford Dictionary 2001). There are significant differences between a child and an adolescent, physically, emotionally, sexually and socially (Knight and Rush 1998). For the purpose of this chapter the following age ranges will be associated with different stages of development:

New born	0–6 weeks
Infant	6 weeks to 1 year
Child	1–10 years
Adolescent	>10 years

It is essential that when caring for children and young people that there is a basic understanding of the developmental stages from infancy through to, and beyond adolescence. Without this underpinning knowledge, assessing the patient accurately is very difficult. As children get older they change in many ways: some distinct and some more discreet.

The terms "growth" and "development" are often used interchangeably; however, it is important to be clear of the differences:

- *Growth* – refers to an increase in size. The course of growth is mainly physical and can be measured with some degree of accuracy in terms of height and weight.
- *Development* – refers to an increase in complexity involving both function and structure (Sheridan 1984).

In emergency care one of the critical pieces of information required to treat a child is their weight. This is essential for working out correct dosages of drugs. We may not have an accurate measure of the child's weight on arrival and their presenting complaint may make weighing them difficult. The following formulae can be applied to estimate the weight (in kg), of a child between the ages of 1–10 years (APLS 2001):

$$\text{Weight (in kg)} = (\text{age (years)} + 4) \times 2$$

It is beyond the scope of this chapter and the remit of this book to cover child development in-depth. Important areas will be highlighted using presenting complaints and considerations under airway, breathing and circulation. For a more in-depth explanation of child development refer to the *Illustrated Textbook of Paediatrics* (Lissauer and Clayden 2001).

NORMAL PHYSIOLOGICAL PARAMETERS FOR CHILDREN AND ADOLESCENTS

AIRWAY

There are key anatomical differences between the paediatric and adult airway with consequences for airway management in the emergency situation (Table 3.1) (APLS 2001).

Infants of less than 6 months are obligate nasal breathers; their narrow nasal passages can become occluded with mucous increasing the risk of airway compromise.

The significance of partial airway obstruction in children cannot be overstated. A small reduction in diameter of the airways can result in a clinically significant increase in airway resistance and therefore increased effort of breathing.

BREATHING

Respiratory illnesses are not uncommon in childhood; however, the consequences for the child can be serious (Wooler 1993). It is well established that cardiac arrest in infants and children is associated with hypoxia (Tunstall and McCarthy 1993; RCN 1998). Therefore, a key step in preventing cardiac arrest is recognition and alleviation of respiratory distress.

Change in the respiratory *rate* and *effort* are crucial indicators of the physical condition of the child and their body's ability to cope with the challenge of the illness or injury.

The normal respiratory rate for different age groups of children is presented in Table 3.2. Respiratory *distress* is a clinical state indicated by a marked increase in the work of breathing. The signs of distress and their clinical relevance are highlighted in Table 3.3.

There are other consequences and effects of increased respiratory effort and the resultant hypoxia or hypercapneoa such as an altered level of consciousness. The AVPU scale (see Chapter 4) is a useful adjunct to this assessment. The parents or individuals accompanying an infant or child will give a guide to their usual mental status. Increasing drowsiness and tiredness are indicators for more aggressive treatment and management. Exhaustion is a pre-terminal sign (APLS 2001). An absence of wheeze, stridor or breath

---

Table 3.1
Key anatomical differences in the infant/child airway (0–10 years) and their consequences

Anatomical difference	Consequence
Narrower airways	Greater risk of obstruction from small amounts of mucous or swelling. Increased airway resistance
Larger tongue	Posterior displacement of the tongue may cause severe obstruction. Can be rectified by proper positioning
Floor of mouth soft	Easily compressed if holding jaw incorrectly
Epiglottis is short and narrow	Acute angle between base of tongue and glottic opening
Trachea is short and soft	Greater risk of compression with over-extension of the neck
Cricoid ring narrowest part of the airway	The cells of the cricoid ring make it particularly susceptible to oedema. The ring provides a natural seal for an uncuffed endotracheal tube. Endotracheal size is determined by the size of cricoid ring

---

Table 3.2
Normal respiratory rate by age

Age	Respiratory rate/minute
Birth–6 weeks	30–60
6 months	25–40
1–2 years	25–35
2–5 years	25–30
5–10 years	20–25
10 years +	15–20

sounds in an individual showing increased respiratory effort is an unwelcome and worrying sign.

A silent chest is a silent killer.

CIRCULATION

The circulating blood volume of a child is less than that of an adult (see Table 3.4). A small fluid loss in a child can represent a large percentage of the total circulating volume and, therefore, have a significant effect on circulatory volume.

Heart rate: The normal physiological response in a child to a decrease in circulatory volume, either through haemorrhage or dehydration, is to increase the heart rate. This is a compensatory mechanism, if circulatory volume is not replaced the heart will be unable to sustain the rate required to perfuse vital organs. Without reversal of the underlying cause, the heart will lose its ability to compensate resulting in bradycardia. Bradycardia in a child is a profoundly worrying sign.

Knowledge of the normal values will assist in the assessment of the circulation (see Table 3.5). However, these physiological markers only present part of the picture, it is essential that physiological measurements (or observations) are interpreted in light of the history. The clinical picture may be worse than it first appears, as the physiological response may provide some temporary compensation for reduced circulatory volume.

Table 3.4
Normal circulating volume

Size	Volume (ml/kg)
Neonate	85–90
Infant	75–80
Child	70–75
Adult	65–70

Table 3.3
Signs and symptoms of respiratory distress and clinical relevance (APLS 2001)

Signs of distress	Relevance
Nasal Flaring	Flaring occurs in inspiration, indicates that the child is trying to draw more air into their lungs
Drooling	May have difficulty in swallowing due to oedema or foreign body, also may be due to the concentration of effort on breathing rather than swallowing
Grunting	Caused by exhalation against partially closed glottis. It can prevent airway collapse at the end of expiration by generating a positive end-expiratory pressure. Sign of severe respiratory distress characteristically in infants
Stridor Wheeze	Usually heard on inspiration; sign of laryngeal or tracheal obstruction Associated with lower airway narrowing and normally on expiration. Degree of wheeze does not correlate with severity. Indeed a silent chest with increased effort may be a pre-morbid sign
Tachypnoea	Indicates an increase in rate to increase ventilation either to increase O_2 or decrease CO_2
Intercostal recession	The tissues between the costal spaces are pulled-in on inspiration. This shows increased work during breathing. The degree or amount of recession gives an indication of the severity of distress
Subcostal recession	The tissues below the costal margins are pulled-in on inspiration. This shows increased work during breathing. The degree or amount of recession gives and indication of the severity of distress
Use of accessory muscles	In infants may present as head bobbing; this is associated with ineffectual breathing. In older children, with more developed sternomastoid muscles the movement of the shoulders will be associated with increased respiratory effort

Table 3.5
Normal circulation parameters

Age	Site	Pulse (bpm)	B/P systolic (mmHg)	Capillary refill (seconds)
Birth–6 weeks	Brachial	100–160	50–95	≤2
6 months–1 year	Brachial	90–160	80–100	≤2
1–2 years	Carotid or radial	90–150	80–100	≤2
2–5 years	Radial	90–140	80–100	≤2
5–10 years	Radial	80–120	90–110	≤2
10 years +	Radial	60–100	90–120	≤2

Table 3.6
Assessment of dehydration (Brown 1999)

	Mild	Moderate	Severe
Percentage of body weight loss	<5%	5–10%	>10%
Appearance	In good general condition	Looks unwell, floppy/ apathetic	Drowsy, cool
Skin condition	Dry mouth and thirst	Sunken fontanelle, dry mouth, decreased skin turgor, marked thirst	Cyanosed
Urine output	Mild oliguria	Oliguria	Anuria
Vital signs	Usually within normal limits	Tachycardia	Tachypnoeic, tachycardic/ bradycardic, hypotensive, may become comatosed risk of sudden death

Level of consciousness: Other indicators of the effectiveness of circulation are level of consciousness/ responsiveness. Alterations in level of consciousness/ responsiveness may be subtle; parental or carer involvements in this assessment (as they have the best knowledge of the child's normal response) as well as careful observation by the nurse are essential.

Capillary refill: Skin perfusion and temperature are also indicators of the effectiveness of circulation to the peripheries. Poor peripheral circulation would be indicated by peripheral cyanosis, skin cool to touch, mottling or pallor and a decreased capillary-refill time. Normal capillary-refill time is ≤2 seconds. It is measured by raising the area to be tested, i.e. the foot or hand, above the level of the heart, pressing on the periphery for 5 seconds and measuring the time it takes for the blanched area (white area) of skin to return to its normal colour. When evaluating capillary-refill

time, you should be aware of the effects of ambient temperature. If the child is exposed to a cold environment, vasoconstriction will result affecting the reliability of the capillary-refill time as a marker of circulatory status. Cosmetics, in the form of nail varnish, may mask changes in the appearance of skin/nails.

Dehydration: Dehydration may be a cause of decreased circulatory volume. As with all assessments the history of illness and injury will raise awareness of dehydration as being a causative factor (such as history of diarrhoea and vomiting). Signs and symptoms of varying degrees of dehydration (see Table 3.6) that may be present are: dry mucous membranes, reduced or absent tears or saliva, loss of skin turgor, sunken eyes (in infants sunken anterior fontanelle), weight loss, altered level of consciousness and tachycardia. Table 3.6 identifies many subjective markers of dehydration. If there is cause for concern consideration should be given to more objective measures such as central venous pressure (CVP) monitoring.

Fluid replacement

Hypovolaemia, whether through trauma or dehydration poses a significant threat to the sick child. Fluid and electrolyte balance is inextricably linked and must be considered when instigating fluid replacement. Previous sections of this chapter have identified normal circulatory parameters and indications of dehydration. When hypovolaemia is suspected, a bolus of intravenous (IV) fluid can be calculated on the basis of 20 ml or crystalloid or colloid per kg of body weight and given by IV push. The child's response to this initial bolus should be assessed, the bolus can be repeated if there is insufficient improvement. After the second bolus, if there is no improvement, a transfusion of blood should be considered (APLS 2001). In the case of dehydration, the child should be assessed for signs of shock, if present then the regime as described for hypovolaemia should be initiated, however, if there are no signs of shock oral re-hydration should be considered. If oral re-hydration is not possible, then an infusion of 0.9% saline should be commenced (APLS 2001). Consideration should be given to hypoglycaemia its correction.

It is beyond the scope of this chapter to discuss the fluid and electrolyte replacement in-depth. For a more in-depth explanation of the fluid balance and electrolyte replacement, see the *Advanced Paediatric Life Support: The practical approach* (APLS 2001).

Assessment

As with other aspects of emergency nursing, one of the key skills and roles in caring for children is that of assessment. This is particularly important with children where the signs and symptoms of illness may not be as marked as in adults. Children are able to compensate for alterations in physiology, but their reserve or ability to sustain that compromise is limited. Careful observation and repeated observations are required to ensure those subtle cues or signs of illness are detected (Alcock et al 2002).

> Assessment is not a singular event, it is a continuous and dynamic process.

The following sections of this chapter will highlight common presentations, their signs and symptoms and approaches to assessment and management.

RESPIRATORY DISTRESS IN CHILDREN

Causes of respiratory distress can be categorized as upper or lower airway:

Upper airway	Lower airway
Croup	Asthma
Epiglottitis	Bronchiolitis
Trauma	Trauma
Aspiration of foreign body	Aspiration of foreign body
Congenital abnormalities	Pneumonia

All respiratory difficulties will cause fear, distress and agitation for both the child and carer. It is, therefore, essential to assess and treat such presentations in a calm re-assuring manner. Visual presentation, breath sounds and vital signs for the most common presentations are presented in Table 3.7. The following sections will outline features of these diseases and the immediate management required.

Acute breathlessness is an extremely frightening experience for both the child and carer. A calm approach and skilful management will aid re-assurance.

Obtaining a good history of the illness and precipitating factors to the child/adolescents attendance is fundamental to assessment.

Record peak flow (if possible) and document decrease from their normal range (if known).

Let the child assume their own airway/body position.

ASTHMA
Definition

The International Paediatric Asthma Consensus Group (1992) suggested the following definition of asthma: "A condition in which episodic wheeze and/or cough occur in a clinical setting where asthma is likely and other, rarer conditions have been excluded."

Asthma is a disease characterized by three key factors, cough, wheeze and shortness of breath. In

Suzanne Knight and Robert Crouch

Emergency care of the child and adolescent

Table 3.7
Typical presentations for different forms of respiratory distress

	Asthma	Bronchiolitis	Croup	Epiglottitis	Aspiration of foreign body
Visual presentation	Cough Short of breath Irritability	Cough Nasal flaring Sternal/intercostals retraction	Barking cough Nasal flaring Hoarse voice Exhaustion Mouth breathing Increased work of breathing	Increased work of breathing Upright forward position known as the "frog position" Open mouth and protruding tongue Drooling	Distressed Drooling Difficulty swallowing Gagging Choking Cough
Breath sounds	Expiratory wheeze Decreased or unequal breath sounds Silent chest in severe cases	Wheezing Grunting	Inspiratory stridor Blocked nose	Expiratory snore Inspiratory stridor	Inspiratory stridor Absent or decreased breath sounds Unilateral wheeze
Vital signs	Abnormal peak flow Tachypnoea	Tachypnoea Apnoea spells Low-grade fever	Low-grade fever Tachycardia Tachypnoea	Pyrexia Tachycardia	Reduced conscious level Loss of colour Signs of asphyxiation Cardio-respiratory arrest

children, the first manifestation may be as a nocturnal cough, which parents may have dismissed as insignificant for some time. The wheeze or cough is as a result of a reduced airway lumen. The mechanisms involved in this include: increased bronchoconstrictor response, oedema and or hypersecretions of mucus (Wong 1999; Wooler 1993).

There are a number of predisposing factors to asthma and its exacerbation which include:

- allergies,
- exercise,
- infections,
- irritants,
- weather changes,
- smoking,
- emotions.

For signs and symptoms of presentation, see Table 3.7.

Assessment

- Airway, breathing and circulation

- Oxygen saturation
- Level of consciousness
- Temperature

Interventions

- Administer high-flow humidified oxygen via a non-rebreather mask.
- Monitor oxygen saturation, respiratory rate and heart rate.
- Support child to adopt an upright position (small children respond best when sat on parents' lap).
- Re-assure both child and carer.
- Keep the child with a parent or familiar adult.
- Pre- and post-peak flow, if the child is able to co-operate.
- Administer nebulized salbutamol 2.5–5 mg (18 months +) diluted to 5 ml with normal saline; add ipratropium (atrovent) 125–250 µg to next salbutamol nebulizer, if initial one is ineffective. (*Note*: salbutamol nebulizers can be given continuously until there is improvement (Brown 1999).)

- Consider IV access depending on severity of attack, consider IV salbutamol.
- Consider oral prednisilone, 1–2 mg/kg (to a maximum of 40 mg), which may shorten the duration of an acute attack and may prevent rebound symptoms.
- Fluids, IV, if the child is unable to drink due to shortness of breath.
- Prepare for admission to paediatric ward.
- Consider IV aminophyline, magnesium.

BRONCHIOLITIS
Definition

Viral infection, most commonly caused by the respiratory syncytial virus (RSV). It occurs usually in infants of less than 1 year of age peaking at 6 months. Commonly the onset is gradual, characterized by a runny nose, cough, vomiting and poor fluid intake. The mechanisms involved include inflammation of the bronchioles and increase secretion of mucous (Brown 1999; ENA 1993).

For signs and symptoms of presentation, see Table 3.7.

Assessment

- Airway, breathing and circulation
- Level of consciousness
- Oxygen saturation
- Temperature

Interventions

- Administer high flow humidified oxygen.
- Monitor oxygen saturation, respiratory rate and heart rate.
- Support the child in the upright position on parents knee if possible.
- Re-assurance for parents and child.
- Assess frequency and characteristic of cough.
- Close observation of respiration and work of breathing, as signs of exhaustion must be recognized immediately and infant/child may have apnoeic episodes. Consider preparation for intubation and ventilation and transfer to ITU.
- Consider IV access.

- Fluid replacement orally, if possible.
- Monitor urine output (in young children, weighing nappies pre- and post-urination may be required).
- Monitor any changes in fontanelles, skin turgor and mucus membranes.
- Admission to a paediatric ward.
- Contact isolation – it is fundamental that the well- being of siblings and close contacts is considered particularly those who may be vulnerable to respiratory illness.

CROUP
Definition

An acute viral respiratory illness, most commonly caused by the parainfluenza virus. It affects boys and girls equally and is the most common in the under 3-year-old-age group. The most frequent presentations are in autumn and winter. The mechanisms involved include inflammation and oedema surrounding the trachea and vocal chords, and the production of thick secretions in the lower respiratory tract. Predisposing factors include exposure to parainfluenza virus or RSV and chest infection.

For signs and symptoms of presentation, see Table 3.7.

Assessment

- Airway, breathing and circulation
- Level of consciousness
- Oxygen saturation
- Temperature

Interventions

- Humidified atmosphere.
- In cases of severe respiratory distress, nebulised adrenaline 5 ml of 1 : 1000 should be considered (NB cardiac monitoring required).
- Support the child in the upright position on parents knee, if possible.
- Re-assurance for child and parent.
- Oral fluids, if tolerated.
- Consider IV access for fluids, if not being taken orally.

- Additional medications as prescribed.
- Monitor oxygen saturation, respiratory rate and heart rate.
- Anti-pyretics measures, if required.

EPIGLOTTITIS
Definition

An acute bacterial infection, commonly caused by the hemophilus influenza type B. Swelling of the epigottis and surrounding tissue causes airway obstruction rapidly. It usually occurs in children aged between 2 and 6 years although it can occur in older children and adults. This is a rare but potentially life-threatening condition.

Characteristics

- Rapid onset
- Sore throat
- Drooling
- Agitation
- Absence of spontaneous cough
- Pyrexia

Do not attempt to examine the child's throat.
Do not lie the child down to examine them.

Assessment

- Airway, breathing and circulation
- Level of consciousness
- Oxygen saturation
- Temperature

Interventions

- Visual inspection of child.
- Keep carer with the child.
- Calm approach.
- Allow child to adopt a position of comfort.
- Deliver O_2 by any method tolerated by child.
- Consider nebulized adrenaline 5 ml 1 : 1000.
- Prepare emergency airway equipment – cricothyroidotomy.

- Prepare for rapid transfer to resuscitation or theatre for intubation (normally gas induction).
- Protect the child from unnecessary examination.
- Ensure senior anaesthetic and ear, nose and throat specialist are present.

ASPIRATION OF FOREIGN BODIES
Definition

This occurs most commonly in children under the age of 5 years and is a major cause of morbidity and mortality in children (Lorin 1990). Epiglottitis should be considered as a differential diagnosis for aspiration of a foreign body. The most commonly aspirated objects include food (e.g. peanuts), coins, batteries, buttons, small toys, etc. The response to aspiration depends on the object and the degree of obstruction. Dry foods such as popcorn will swell as they come into contact with the mucous membranes, thus adding further complications (Carter 1995).

Characteristics

- Acute onset of symptoms, occurring during or immediately after activities such as playing or eating.
- History of gagging, refusing to eat or vomiting.

Mechanisms involved

- Localized inflammation of upper/lower respiratory tract.
- Partial or total occlusion of the airway.

Assessment

- Airway, breathing and circulation
- Level of consciousness
- Oxygen saturation

Interventions

If the child appears to be choking or deteriorating, instigate Resuscitation Council (UK) 2000 guidelines techniques for choking (p. 35).

- The priority is to clear the airway.
- Provide supplementary oxygen as required.
- Call for medical help.
- Otherwise, keep the child and carer calm.
- Nurse in a quiet, relaxed atmosphere.
- Refer appropriate speciality, i.e. ear, nose and throat.
- Prepare for bronchoscopy.

GUIDELINES FOR CHOKING
Infant (conscious)

1 Hold the child on your forearm, with his face down, supporting the head by firmly holding the jaw. Rest your forearm on your leg. The infant's body must be lower than his trunk.
2 Deliver up to five back blows between the infants shoulders, using the heal of your hand.
3 Supporting the infant, turn him over, whilst supporting the head so that he is in a supine position, again, the head must be lower than the trunk.
4 Give up to five quick downward chest thrusts (two fingers on the lower half of the sternum, one finger's breadth below the nipple line).

Repeat these steps until the foreign body is removed or the infant loses consciousness, in which case follow the next steps.

Infant (unconscious)

1 Open the airway, using the tongue–chin lift remove the foreign body, if you can see it (never perform a blind finger sweep).
2 Attempt up to five rescue breaths to achieve two effective breaths.
3 If unsuccessful, reposition the child.
4 If ventilation is again unsuccessful, give five back blows and five chest thrusts.
5 Repeat step 1.
6 Repeat steps 2–5 until ventilation is successful.

Child (conscious)

If the child is breathing spontaneously, encourage his own efforts to clear the airway. Intervention is only necessary if this is ineffective and breathing is inadequate.

1 Hold the child in a prone position, attempt to keep the head lower than the chest, with the airway in an open position.
2 Give up to five smart blows to the middle of the back between the shoulder blades.
3 If unsuccessful, turn the child into a supine position, again with the head lower than the chest and with the airway open.
4 Give up to five chest thrusts to the sternum (these are similar to chest compressions, but sharper and more vigorous).
5 Check mouth and carefully remove any visible foreign bodies.

Child (unconscious)

1 Lay the child in a supine position.
2 Attempt up to five rescue breaths to achieve two effective breaths.
3 Repeat the cycles 1–5 as above, but substitute five abdominal thrusts for the five chest compressions (abdominal thrusts should be delivered as five sharp thrusts directed upward towards the diaphragm).
4 Alternate chest thrusts and abdominal thrusts in subsequent cycles.
5 Repeat cycles until the airway is clear or the child breathes spontaneously.

(Resuscitation Council (UK) 2000)

The following sections will deal with a number of life-threatening conditions and common presentations to the Emergency Department.

BACTERIAL MENINGITIS
Definition

An acute infection of the meninges and cerebro-spinal fluid (CSF), most frequently affecting children aged between 1 month and 5 years (Wong 1999) can affect any child or adolescent of any age. Bacterial meningitis continues to have a mortality rate of more than 5%, with a similar rate of serious or permanent neurological damage (Morton et al 1996).

Suzanne Knight and Robert Crouch

Characteristics

- Headache
- Fever
- Neck stiffness*
- Photophobia*

Mechanisms involved

- Inflammation of meninges
- Inflammation of CSF
- Raised intracranial pressure (ICP)

Predisposing factors

- Exposure to bacterial agent (Haemophilus influenzae, Meningococcus and Streptococcus pneumoniae)
- Deficiencies in the immune system
- Pre-existing CNS anomalies
- Sickle cell disease

          (Wong 1995; Morton and Phillips 1996)

The signs and symptoms for infants/young children and children/adolescents are presented in Table 3.8.

Assessment

- Airway, breathing and circulation
- Level of consciousness
- Oxygen saturation
- Temperature
- Examine skin for rash
- Blood glucose

Interventions

Any child who is unwell and has developed a purpuric rash must be assessed immediately by a doctor.

This is an exceptionally worrying and frightening time for both the carer and child, clear and honest explanations along with a calm approach are essential.

---

*These classic characteristics are often absent, or are difficult to judge in an irritable young child. Older children and adolescents are easier to assess, their symptoms often being more abrupt (Morton et al 1996).

Table 3.8
Signs and symptoms for bacterial meningitis

Infants and young children	Children and adolescents
Drowsiness	Drowsiness
Lack of eye contact with parents	Altered conscious level
Pyrexia	Coma
Vomiting	Often abrupt onset
Poor feeding	Headache
Irritability	Fever
Convulsions	Vomiting
Apnoea	Agitation
Cyanosis	Irritability
Purpuric rash	Aggressive behaviour
High-pitched cry	Photophobia
Bulging fontanel	Neck stiffness
Rigidity	Petechial or purpuric rash

- Administer high-flow oxygen (elevated temperature increases the brain's metabolic and oxygen needs).
- IV access* (if time allows apply local anaesthetic cream to areas suitable for IV access).
- Antibiotic therapy*.
- Bloods – U&Es, creatinine, magnesium, calcium, clotting screen, group and save, and blood cultures.
- IV fluids as required.
- Monitor vital signs, including temperature and neurological status.
- If possible nurse the child in a quiet, darkened environment (to reduce noxious stimuli).
- Analgesia/anti-pyretics (to reduce pain and pyrexia, thus reducing the chances of the child fitting).
- Paediatric referral.
- Prepare for admission.

---

* If the child has a purpuric rash, instigate immediately.

ASEPTIC (VIRAL/FUNGAL) MENINGITIS

Definition

Principally a viral infection of the meninges, associated with a number of childhood diseases such as measles, mumps, herpes and leukaemia. This usually occurs in children over the age of two. Onset may be abrupt or gradual. Symptoms generally subside spontaneously within 3–10 days, with no residual effect (Wong 1999; Morton 1996).

Characteristics

- Photophobia
- Headache
- Neck stiffness
- Vomiting

NB Children presenting with aseptic meningitis are less ill than those with bacterial.

Mechanisms involved

- Irritation of the meninges due to a viral/fungal infection.

Predisposing factors

- Measles
- Mumps
- Herpes
- Leukaemia
- Enteric organisms

Signs and symptoms

- Headache
- Photophobia
- General malaise
- Abdominal pain
- Back and leg pain
- Vomiting
- Sore throat
- Fever
- Maculopapular rash
- Neck stiffness

NB In infants and toddlers the onset of symptoms is more insidious. Parents may report changes in the child's responsiveness and level of activity (Wong 1999). Not all the signs and symptoms need to be present to diagnose meningitis.

Assessment

- Airway, breathing and circulation
- Level of consciousness
- Oxygen saturation
- Temperature
- Examine skin for rash
- Blood glucose

Interventions

- Administer oxygen as required.
- IV access (if time allows apply local anaesthetic cream to areas suitable for IV access).
- Monitor vital signs, including temperature.
- Monitor conscious level.
- Anti-pyretics.
- Analgesics.
- Comfortable positioning.
- Prepare for admission.

FEBRILE CONVULSION

Definition

A transient neurological disorder of a child that is associated with a fever. Febrile convulsions are the most common neurologic disorders of childhood. They usually occur between the ages of 6 months and 3 years, with an increased frequency in those under 18 months. They take place twice as often in boys as in girls, there appears to be a genetic predisposition, with an increased susceptibility in families (Wong 1999). Before the age of 5 years, between 2% and 4% of all children in Europe and the USA will experience at least one convulsion associated with a fever (Hausser 1994).

Characteristics

- Febrile child
- Generalized tonic-clonic event

- "Funny turn"
- Frightened parents

Serious consideration to the possibility of meningitis as a differential diagnosis, should be given to every child who presents with a febrile convulsion.

Mechanisms involved

- Cause remains uncertain
- Elevated temperature

Predisposing factors

- Upper respiratory tract infection
- Gastro-intestinal infection
- Recent immunisations
- Otitis media
- Urinary tract infection
- Pneumonia

Signs and symptoms

- Reduced level of consciousness
- Tonic-clonic limb movements
- Pyrexia
- Tachycardia
- Tachypnoena
- Lethargy
- Irritability

Assessment

- Airway, breathing and circulation
- Level of consciousness
- Oxygen saturation
- Temperature
- Blood glucose
- Urinalysis

Interventions

Most children who have had a febrile convulsion will have stopped fitting by the time they reach the ED.

If fitting on arrival, follow the fitting protocol outlined in the next section.

- Give supplementary oxygen.
- Remove excess clothing (keep cotton vest on).
- Record temperature.
- Administer weight-related dose of anti-pyretics.
- Record pulse and respiration.
- Re-assure parents, who may be extremely frightened.
- Use fan to cool child (not too high a setting).
- Reassess temperature.
- Prepare for admission as per hospital protocol.

THE FITTING CHILD

Call for senior medical assistance.

- Maintain the airway (consider nasal airway).
- Suction any secretions from the mouth.
- Administer high-flow oxygen.
- Nurse the child on his/her side with head tipped downwards.
- Assist in gaining IV access.
- Administer anticonvulsant as per policy.
- Monitor blood glucose.
- Get a full set of vital signs, including oxygen saturation and neurological observations.
- Monitor vital signs at 15 minute intervals.
- Re-assure parents/careers.
- Keep the child safe, using cot sides, if necessary.
- Assist with blood sampling.
- Prepare for admission.
- Do not give food or liquids until fully alert and swallowing reflex has returned.

ALTERED STATE OF CONSCIOUSNESS

Definition

Varying states of consciousness can range from momentary to indefinite. *Consciousness* indicates the ability to respond to sensory stimuli (alertness) and the ability to process stimuli producing verbal and motor responses (cognitive power). *Unconsciousness* is a depressed cerebral function. *Coma* is a state of unconsciousness, from which the patient cannot be aroused (Wong 1999).

Suzanne Knight and Robert Crouch

Characteristics

- Confusion
- Disorientation
- Lethargy
- Obtundation (arousable with stimulation)
- Stupor (responsive only to vigorous stimulation)
- Coma

Mechanisms involved

- Impairment of the reticular formation in the brain

Predisposing factors

- Infections (i.e. bacterial meningitis, viral encephalitis)
- Fluid loss (i.e. hypovolaemia in severe gastro-enteritis)
- Trauma
- Head injury
- Poisoning (including alcohol)
- Metabolic conditions (diabetes)

(Morton et al 1996)

Signs and symptoms

- Inappropriate eye-opening response
- Confusion
- Disorientation
- Altered motor response
- Aggressiveness
- Drowsy
- Agitation
- Persistent crying
- Restless
- Combative
- Sleepy
- Lethargic

NB When considering signs and symptoms, it is important to have an understanding of the developmental stages in children. For example, the best response to auditory ± visual stimulus for a child over 2 years may be "orientated", whereas for a child under 2 years, the best response may be "smiles, listens, follows".

Assessment

- Airway, breathing and circulation
- Level of consciousness
- Oxygen saturation
- Temperature
- Examine skin for rash
- Look for signs of trauma
- Blood glucose
- Urinalysis

Interventions

- Administer high-flow oxygen.
- Record neurological status, using an assessment chart that is appropriate to the child's age.
- Assess and record coma scale.
- Record and control temperature.
- Record pulse, respiration and blood pressure.
- Monitor neurological signs at 15–30 minute intervals.
- Record blood glucose, if less than 3 mmol/l inform medical team and administer dextrose (5 ml/kg of 10% dextrose).
- Position on side.
- Get a full history of the event leading to the child's current condition.
- Identify possible drugs taken and contact nearest poisons unit.
- Involve parents/carers when performing neurological observations as the child may respond better to them.
- Re-assure and comfort parents/carers.
- If necessary, prepare for admission.

Occasionally children, especially adolescents may try to feign unconsciousness; this can become apparent by the lack of genuine physical signs. In such cases, referral to a counselling service may be required for underlying behavioural/social or psychological problems (Morton et al 1996).

DIARRHOEA AND VOMITING

Definition

Diarrhoea and vomiting (D&V) is one of the most common problems experienced by infants and young children. Diarrhoea has been defined as increased stool production or a decrease in the consistency of the stool, which leads to fluid loss. It can have profound physiological effects upon the child and is potentially life threatening (Smith 1988). Most children are nursed at home with this condition. In the UK, it is likely that those who attend the ED will be under 2 years of age (Dearman et al 1995).

Characteristics

- Progressive diarrhoea
- Vomiting
- Unable to tolerate fluids
- Reduced urine output
- Apathy

Mechanisms involved

- Loss of sodium through vomiting.
- Loss of potassium through diarrhoea.
- Shift of intracellular fluid compartments to extracellular compartments.
- Alterations in acid–base balance.

Predisposing factors

- Infections
- Poor sterilizing techniques
- Food contamination
- Allergy
- Food sensitivity (Khatib 1986)
- Metabolic abnormalities
- Intercerception/bowel obstruction

Signs and symptoms

- Sunken eyes
- Sunken fontanelles
- Poor skin elasticity/turgor
- Cold extremities
- Tachycardia
- Hypotension
- Reduced urine output
- Vomiting
- Unable to tolerate fluids
- Diarrhoea
- Irritable
- Apathetic
- Pale/cyanosed
- Pyrexia

Assessment

- Airway, breathing and circulation
- Level of consciousness
- Oxygen saturation
- Temperature
- Examine skin for rash
- Blood glucose
- Urinalysis/stool cultures inspect for blood
- Check for signs and symptoms of dehydration (see Table 3.5).

Interventions

> If the child is exhibiting signs of hypovolaemia, seek urgent medical attention.

- Monitor vital signs.
- Give oral rehydration fluids, avoid milk products.
- Initiate IV infusion in severe cases or naso-gastric tube feeding.
- Monitor urine output (weigh wet nappies).
- Get a stool sample.
- Prepare for admission, if required.

TOXICOLOGICAL EMERGENCIES

Definition

"Poisoning" refers to the occurrence of a chemical injury to a body system(s). Suspected poisoning in children accounts for 40,000 Emergency Department attendance's each year in England (Morton et al 1996).

Characteristics

Characteristics depend largely on what has been ingested.

- Frequently there are no immediate ill effects
- Evidence of substance ingested (i.e. smell of domestic substance on clothes)
- Burns around and in the mouth
- Pinpoint pupils (opiates)
- Dilated pupils (atropine compounds)
- Confusion/excitability (alcohol, solvent abuse, dexamphetamine)

Mechanisms involved

Characteristically, poisoning occurs through one of five routes:

- oral,
- dermal,
- ocular,
- inhalation,
- IV injection.

The most common products ingested by children include:

- detergents,
- plants,
- household products,
- medication,
- vitamins.

Predisposing factors

- *Intentional* (by child or an adult knowingly overdosing a child)
- Social/psychological problems
- Experimental
- *Unintentional/accidental*
- Unsupervised child
- Experimental

Signs and symptoms

- Vary with each toxicological emergency
- Positive/possible history
- Airway obstruction
- Cough
- Stridor
- Breathing difficulties
- Reduced level of consciousness
- Rash
- Pinpoint/dilated pupils
- Cardiac arrhythmias
- Confusion
- Anxiety
- Tachycardia
- Excitability
- Ataxia
- Hypotension
- Hypertension

Assessment

- Airway, breathing and circulation
- Level of consciousness
- Oxygen saturation
- Temperature
- Examine skin for rash/burns
- Blood glucose
- Use sense of smell

Interventions

The symptoms of poisoning will vary considerably depending on the type, amount and quantity of toxins involved. It is, therefore, essential that a swift assessment be made.

- A thorough history must be taken to include:
  - possible toxin,
  - time of ingestion,
  - route of ingestion,
  - description of subsequent symptoms.
- Obtain information from local source of poisons information either via the world wide web (www) or via telephone for management and treatment of the identified toxin.
- Monitor conscious level, respiratory rate and depth, and pulse rate.
- Blood pressure.
- Pupil size and reactivity.
- Observe skin and mouth for evolving contact burns.
- Give activated charcoal according to the child's weight, if appropriate.
- Provide support for family/carer who may feel they are to blame.
- Instigate local child protection procedures, if the poisoning is thought to be intentional by an adult.
- Prepare child for admission, if required.
- Contact social worker/child psychologist, if required.
- Health promotion and accident prevention, if required.

INGESTION OF ALCOHOL

Definition

Children of all ages ingest alcohol. For the younger age range, this is usually accidental; however, this is not always the case for older children. Adolescents often experiment with alcohol; it is one of the commonest forms of drug abuse in this age range in the UK (Morton et al 1996).

Signs and symptoms

The clinical features are similar to those in adults and are dependent upon the amount ingested and the individual's tolerance. For children only a small amount of alcohol needs to be ingested to produce symptoms:

- feeling of warmth, cheerfulness,
- impairment of judgement,
- loss of inhibition,
- slurred speech,
- double vision,
- memory loss,
- ataxia,
- vomiting,
- loss of consciousness.

Many of these signs and symptoms can be associated with other presentations such as raised intercranial pressure and hypoglycaemia.

> Be careful that your assessment and care is not compromised by a judgement that this is just alcohol.

Assessment

- Airway, breathing and circulation
- Level of consciousness
- Oxygen saturation
- Temperature
- Examine skin for rash/sings of injury
- Blood glucose

> Children easily develop hypoglycaemia and hypothermia with alcohol ingestion.

Interventions

- Prevent aspiration of vomit.
- Give oral/IV fluids.
- Obtain a social/psychiatric history.
- Raise a concern with school nurse/social worker.

- Health promotion.
- Possible referral to counselling service.

The following section will deal with three challenging issues in paediatric emergency care dealing with sudden infant death syndrome, child protection and abuse through prostitution.

SUDDEN INFANT DEATH

Sudden infant death (SID) or cot death has been defined as "the sudden and unexpected death of a baby for no obvious reason" (Foundation for the Study of Infant Deaths (FSID) 1997). In the UK, this is the most prevalent category of death in infants between the ages of 1 month and 1 year (FSID 1997), with a majority of SIDs (80%) occurring under 6 months of age (RCN 1998). Many theories have been suggested regarding the aetiology of SID, but the exact cause remains unknown (Wong 1999).

Dealing with an SID can be distressing for all involved. However, management of this in a sympathetic and confident manner can help parents come to terms with the loss of their baby (RCN 1998).

If they wish to be present in the resuscitation room, the parent(s) should be allowed to remain with their child, but must be supported by a nurse (RCN 1998). If the parent(s) do not wish to be there, they should be taken to a private room, which is comfortable, has access to a telephone and is reserved exclusively for their use (RCN 1998; Morton 1996). A nurse must be allocated to care for the relatives. Although it is important to remain with them, the nurse needs be sensitive to the fact that they may value time alone. If they wish so, the services of a minister of their particular religion should be offered.

Following confirmation of the baby's death, it may be appropriate for the professional who has had the most contact with the relatives to break the "bad news". Prior to this, make sure that the baby's name is known to those breaking this news. It is important that staff sit at the same level as the parents and that information is given in a sympathetic manner, but without the use of euphemisms. At some point the parents will ask the reason for their child's death, answer as simply and honestly.

When the parent(s) are ready, a full history of events will be required; the parents will require considerable support. The parent(s) will need to be informed that all sudden and unexplained deaths must be reported to a coroner and that this usually takes the form of a Police Officer attending to ask them questions. A post-mortem will be required to determine the cause of death, naturally the thought of this can be extremely distressing. Re-assurance should be given that the child will be handled carefully and that a post-mortem is like an operation after death (Morton and Phillips 1996). It is also necessary that they understand why a post-mortem is required.

The parent(s) should be allowed as much time as they require with their child. If possible, the child should remain in his or her own clothes, unless they are soiled, in which case appropriate clothes kept in the department should be used.

The taking of mementoes and photographs has been shown to assist parents in the grieving process. These provide confirmation of their child's existence in infancy and act as a lasting memory (Osborne 2000). Hand- and foot-prints, photographs and hair lockets can be taken with the parent's consent and placed in a "book of keepsakes". The parent(s) may be too distressed to take this straightaway, if this is the case the booklet should either be kept in the child's notes or in a designated place in the department. The parent(s) should be informed that if they so wish, this can be collected at a time convenient to them.

A departmental checklist containing the following information is a useful tool to ensure that no details have been forgotten:

Child's name	
Date of birth	
Date of death	
Doctor has spoken to the parents	Y/N
Paediatric Registrar/Consultant informed	Y/N
Coroner informed	Y/N
Brief clinical history taken	Y/N
Parents offered to be with/hold baby	Y/N
General Physician (GP) informed	Y/N
Health Visitor informed	Y/N
Post-mortem investigations taken (blood, urine, skin samples and nasal swab)	Y/N
Minister of religion contacted	Y/N
Mementoes/photographs taken	Y/N
Mementoes taken by parents?	Y/N

Information re: post-mortem given	Y/N
Advise on registration and funeral given	Y/N
Pamphlet from FSID given	Y/N
Social worker informed, if required	Y/N
Surviving twin seen by paediatricians	Y/N
Medical records informed and existing appointments cancelled	Y/N
Advise re: breast-feeding	Y/N
Child protection nurse specialist informed	Y/N
Child's body labelled	Y/N
	(RCN 1998; Morton and Phillips 1996)

If the mother has been breast-feeding, she may wish to have a lactation suppressant prescribed, this can be obtained from her GP. If there is a surviving twin, they are at an increased risk (if SID) and should be referred to the paediatric department (Morton and Phillips 1996).

Managing an SID can be extremely stressful for all the team, including the ambulance crew and police officers. It is crucial that time is set aside to reflect on the incident and discuss any issues that arise.

CHILD PROTECTION

Child protection has been defined as "the promotion of decisive action to protect children from abuse and neglect" (Home Office et al 1991). The National Commission into the prevention of child abuse (1996) states:

Child abuse consists of anything which individuals, institutions or processes do or fail to do which directly harms children or damages their prospects of a safe and healthy development into adulthood.

Emergency nurses have a vital role in recognizing and responding to situations that may be indicative of actual, likely or frequent abuse or neglect. The nurse must be proactive in prevention, early detection of family dysfunction and provide support (Powell 1997).

Types of abuse

- Physical (non-accidental injury)
- Sexual

Suzanne Knight and Robert Crouch

- Neglect (psycho-social depravation)
- Non-accidental poisoning
- Suffocation
- Munchausen syndrome by proxy

The primary role of the nurse is to express a "concern" rather than make a "diagnosis" (Swann 1993). Concerns about a child must always be made known to a senior nurse and doctor.

Possible behavioural and physical indicators of abuse

It may include:

- Multiple bruising, soft tissue injuries
- Multiple fractures, fractures in children under 3 years
- Burns
- Adult bite marks
- Failure to thrive
- Torn frenulum
- Excessive sadness
- Frozen watchfulness
- Self-mutilation
- Overdose
- Indiscriminate attachment
- Precocious sexual activity
- Pregnancy
- Sexually transmitted disease
- Genital or rectal bleeding

(Powell 1997)

These indicators are not definitive and must be taken in context with other factors. Considerations such as repeated attendance, delay in attendance, a mismatch in between the injury and the explanation for the injury and poor family dynamics must be taken into account. In order to make an accurate assessment the clinician assessing the child requires a basic understanding of child development in order to consider if the presenting complaint is congruous with the child's developmental stage, i.e. bruising to a non-mobile baby.

Any concerns about a child must always be reported to the nurse-in-charge and senior doctor, who will decide whether to activate the agreed child protection policy. If the concerns do not warrant a specific child protection referral, they should be made known to the departmental liaison health visitor and social worker.

All children attending the ED should be checked against the child protection register. If they are on the register, the senior nurse should investigate whether the presenting complaint is consistent with the reason for registration, if so, a child protection referral should be made.

All departments must have an agreed policy for management of child protection incidents, including skin maps and non-accidental injury checklists.

SEXUALLY EXPLOITED CHILDREN

Child prostitution is an under-researched and poorly understood area of child protection (Linehan 1997; Barrette and Bequeath 1996). Worldwide, an estimated 10 million children are victims of today's sex industry (Hecht 1997). Twelve-year-old girls are being abused through prostitution in the UK (Barnardos 1997). Coerced or lured into prostitution, children are denied their rights, dignity and childhood (Department of Health (DoH) 2000). It is vital to note that this is an issue for boys as well as girls. The importance of early recognition and understanding of this form of abuse cannot be overemphasized (Linehan 1997); the DoH (2000) assert that all professionals must be able to recognize situations where children are involved or are at risk of becoming involved in prostitution.

Definition

Child prostitution has been defined as "the provision of sexual services in exchange for some form of payment such as money, drugs drink or even a bed or roof over one's head" (Green 1992).

Common factors leading to abuse through prostitution

- History of abuse, predominately sexual
- Children who run away from home
- Children in care
- Children with a low self-esteem and poor self-image
- Vulnerable children who are looking for love, affection and a sense of belonging

(DoH 2000; Barrette 1999; Barnardos 1997)

Suzanne Knight and Robert Crouch

Indicators

These indicators should not be viewed as conclusive and must be taken into context with other factors. However, they should raise suspicion (Southampton Area Child Protection Committee (SACPC) 2001):

- Accompanied to the department by an adult (usually male) who is significantly older (>5 years).
- Strong attachment by the accompanying adult (a reluctance to leave the child).
- The adult appearing to maintain "control" of the child.
- Reports from a reliable source that the child has been seen in places known to be used for prostitution.
- Recent episodes of running away, going missing, staying out overnight without plausible explanation.
- Wearing clothes associated with prostitution.
- Carrying large sums of money without plausible explanation.
- Looking well cared for despite no known base.
- Drug/alcohol misuse.
- Self-harm.
- Sexually transmitted diseases/infections.
- Request for contraception advice or services.

If there are any concerns about a child they should be discussed with the named professional (DoH 2000) or directly with Social Services.

If a child is identified as being abused through prostitution, the agreed local child protection policy must be activated.

Agencies to contact

Nurses need to be aware of the local agencies who can advise on this form of abuse.

- Named professionals (see local guidelines).
- Social services.
- Child protection nurse specialist.
- Outreach workers.

In order to ensure uniformity of care for these children, departmental guidelines that are based on an inter-agency approach should be developed.

CONCLUSION

Children and adolescents form a significant proportion of the workload in the ED. Effective assessment and management of the child requires particular skills and knowledge. This chapter has provides an introduction to these.

References

Advanced Paediatric Life Support – The practical approach (2001) 3rd ed. London: BMJ Publishing Group.

Alcock K, Clancy M, Crouch R (2002) Physiological observations of patients admitted from A&E. *Nurs Stand* 8: 33–37.

American Heart Association (1998) *Pediatric advanced life support.* Dallas: American Heart Association.

Berg A (1993) Are febrile seizures provoked by a rapid rise in temperature? *Am J Dis Child* 143: 25–27.

Barnardos (1997) *Who's daughter next?* London: Barnardos.

Barrett D (1999) Reaching out to child prostitutes. *Nurs Stand* 13(13): 22–23.

Barrett D, Beckett W (1996) Child prostitution: reaching out to children who sell sex to survive. *Br J Nurs* 5(18): 1120–1123.

Brown A (1999) *Accident and emergency diagnosis and management* 3rd ed. Oxford: Butterworth-Heinemann.

Carter B (1995) Nursing support and care: meeting the needs of the child and family with altered respiratory function. In: Carter B, Dearmun A, eds. *Child health care nursing.* Oxford: Blackwell Science.

Dearman A, Campbell S, Barlow J (1995) Nursing support and care: meeting the needs of the child and family with altered gastro-intestinal function. In: Carter B, Dearman A, eds. *Child health care nursing.* Oxford: Blackwell Science.

Department of Health (2000) *Safeguarding children involved in prostitution.* London: The Stationary Office.

Foundation for the Study of Infant Deaths (1997) *Sudden infant death: a workbook for professionals.* London: Foundation for the Study of Infant Death.

Green J (1992) *It's no game.* Leicester: National Youth Agency.

Hausser W (1994) The prevalence and incidents of convulsive disorders in children. *Epilepsia* 35 (Suppl 2) 51–56.

Hecht M (1997) *The world congress against the commercial exploitation of children* (online) 15 February 2001, www.hri.ca/children/texts/wcacsec.shtml

Hill S, Miller C, Kosnik E, Hunt W (1984) Pediatric spinal injuries: a clinical study. *J Neurosurg* (57) 114–129. In: American Heart Association (1997) *Pediatric life support.* Dallas: American Heart Association.

Home Office, Department of Health, Welsh Office et al (1991) *Working together under the Children act 1989: A guide to arrangements for interagency co-operation for the protection of children from abuse.* London: HMSO.

International Paediatric Asthma Consensus Group (1992) follow up statement. *Archiv Dis Child* 67: 240–248.

Khatib H (1986) Acute gastro-enteritis in infants. *Nurs Times* 23 April: 31–32.

Knight S, Rush H (1998) Adolescence: the forgotten factor. *Emergen Nurs* 4(6): 22–29.

Kraus J, Fife D, Conroy C (1987) Pediatric brain injuries: the nature, clinical course, and early outcomes in a defined United States population. *Pediatrics* 79: 501–507.

Linehan T (1997) Who cares? *Nurs Times* 93(22): 22–25.

Lissauer T, Clayden G (2001) *Illustrated textbook of paediatrics* 2nd ed. Edinburgh: Mosby International Limited.

Lorin M (1990) Foreign bodies. In: Oshi F, Deangelis C, Feigin R, Warshaw J, eds. *Principles and practice of pediatrics*, 1348–1350. Philadelphia: Lippincott.

Morton R, Phillips B (1996) *Accidents and emergencies in children*, 2nd ed. Oxford: Oxford University Press.

Muller D et al (1992) *Nursing children: psychology, research and practice*. London: Chapman & Hall.

National Commission Inquiry into the Prevention of Child Abuse (1996) *Childhood matters*. London: The Stationary Office.

Osborne M (2000) Photograph and mementoes, the emergency nurse's role following sudden infant death. *Emergen Nurs* 9(7): 23–25.

Pearsall J (2001) In: Judy Pearsall, ed. *The Concise Oxford Dictionary* 10th ed. revised. Oxford: Oxford University Press.

Powell C (1997) Protecting children in the accident and emergency department. *Accident Emergen Nurs* 5: 76–80.

Royal College of Nursing Children in A&E special interest group (1998) *Nursing children in the accident and emergency department* 2nd ed. London: RCN.

Sheridan M (1984) *From Birth to five years childrens developmental progress* Winsor. Nfer – Nelson.

Smith LG (1988) Home treatment of mild, acute diarrhoea and secondary dehydration of infants and small children: an education programme for parents in a shelter for the homeless. *J Profess Nurs* 4(1): 60–63.

Southampton Area Child Protection Committee (2001) *Local protocol, safeguarding children involved in prostitution.* Southampton: Southampton Area Child Protection Committee.

Swann A (1993) *Recognising abuse.* In: Owen H, Pritchard J. eds. *Good practice in child protection.* London: Jessica Kingsley.

Templeton J (1993) *Mechanisms of injury: biomechanics.* In: Eichelberger M, ed. *Pediatric trauma.* St Louis: Mosby Year Book 20–36.

Tunstall A, McCarthy C (1993) Care of the child with cardiovascular problems. In: Carter B, ed. *Manual of paediatric intensive care nursing.* London: Chapman & Hall.

Wong D (1999) *Nursing care of infants and children* 6th ed. St Louis: Mosby.

Wooler E (1994) On course for knowledge. *Nurs Times* 90(15): 42–44.

Emergency care of the child and adolescent

4 | Emergency care of the adult

Ruth Endacott

This chapter addresses common acute adult presentations to the Emergency Department; for example, asthma or an acute abdomen, commonly referred to as "medical" and "surgical" emergencies.

The chapter is structured around assessment of body systems and patient symptoms. Each section provides an overall *assessment and immediate intervention* box related to general symptoms, to enable prompt recognition and action. The chapter then provides more specific assessment and interventions related to specific diagnoses. Some aspects of assessment are repeated in other chapters, to avoid the reader having to continually cross-reference. As emergency nurses may have to manage the patient over a period of some hours, this chapter takes emergency care beyond the immediate actions on presentation at the Emergency Department.

The main emphasis of this chapter is on assessment and intervention for adults presenting with an acute illness; however, it is important that nurses approach the management of such patients with an index of suspicion for significant illness. The management of trauma injury is addressed in Chapter 7 (Emergency care of the trauma patient).

Key principles underpinning emergency management of the adult patient

- Prompt and comprehensive assessment is essential in order to assimilate information beyond the obvious symptoms described by the patient.
- The importance of gaining information from the family, others present and the person who transported the patient to the Emergency Department (for example, ambulance crew, paramedics) is emphasized.
- Have a high index of suspicion that the patient may have other pre-existing medical problems that he or his family may not report until later.
- Remember the complex inter-relationship between body systems; respiratory problems may, in fact, be a late indicator of cardiac pathology.

RESPIRATORY EMERGENCIES

INITIAL RESPIRATORY ASSESSMENT

The purpose of respiratory assessment is to determine the adequacy of gas exchange (oxygenation of tissues and excretion of carbon dioxide).

It is helpful to consider the transfer of oxygen from the atmosphere to tissue beds as a four stage journey (see Table 4.1); this is useful in pinpointing the cause of any inadequacy in tissue oxygenation (Endacott and Jenks 1997).

VISUAL ASSESSMENT OF RESPIRATION

1 *Rate and depth of respiration* are best assessed following removal of upper clothing, enabling evaluation of respiratory effort and symmetry. The depth of respiration is controlled in an involuntary manner by the respiratory centre but may also be controlled voluntarily by the patient. Shallow respiration may therefore be due to abdominal pain or distension (reducing the movement of the

Emergency care of the adult

Table 4.1
Identifying problems with tissue oxygenation

Stage of oxygen transport	Potential problems	Causes
1 The movement of oxygen into the alveoli (alveolar ventilation)	Reduced airway diameter	■ Airway blockage (sputum plugs; vomit; blood; foreign body) ■ Broncho-constriction ■ Pulmonary oedema
	Inadequate respiratory rate/depth	■ Loss of subatmospheric pressure in intrapleural space (pneumothorax) ■ Reduced movement of diaphragm (paralysis arising from C3, 4 or 5 spinal cord damage; abdominal pain or injuries) ■ Inappropriate stimulation of central and peripheral chemoreceptors (change in blood pH/CO_2; damage or depression of medulla oblongata in brain, for example, drugs or alcohol, or cerebral incident)
	Reduction in available oxygen	■ Smoke inhalation ■ Chemical inhalation
2 Transfer of oxygen across the alveolar capillary membrane	Reduced surface area in alveoli for gas exchange	■ Infection ■ Pulmonary oedema
	Inadequate pulmonary circulation[1]	■ Chest trauma ■ Pulmonary embolism
3 Transport of oxygen on the haemoglobin molecule (oxygen saturation – SaO_2)	Inadequate plasma oxygen[2] (PaO_2) Inadequate haemoglobin	■ May be caused by any of the above ■ Anaemia ■ Carbon monoxide poisoning
4 Movement of oxygen from the haemoglobin to the tissues	Reduced dissociation of oxygen from haemoglobin at the tissues	■ Lowered body temperature[3] ■ Lowered PaO_2 ■ Rise in blood pH (alkalosis)
	Increased diffusion distance	■ Tissue oedema
	Reduced tissue blood supply	■ Local injury ■ Vascular disease

[1]This can be further assessed with the use of a V:Q scan which provides information about the ventilation (V) and perfusion (Q) of lung tissue.
[2]In order for oxygen to bind with haemoglobin (recorded as oxygen saturation or SaO_2), an adequate PaO_2 is required. This is particularly marked when the PaO_2 falls below 8 kPa and is demonstrated on the oxygen haemoglobin dissociation curve.
[3]Hence when several units of blood are required, a blood warmer should be used; a large transfusion of cold blood will actually decrease delivery of oxygen to the tissues.

diaphragm) or chest pain, caused by trauma, infection or ischaemia in the heart or lungs.

Observe chest movements – are they symmetrical? are accessory muscles being used? How much effort is the patient using to breathe? Accessory muscles enhance chest expansion during exercise but are not normally used during normal, quiet breathing. Use of accessory muscles (sternocleidomastoid muscles

in the neck, intercostals, abdominals) whilst the patient is at rest indicates respiratory insufficiency.

In assessing respiratory effort, observe exhalation. If the patient is working hard to exhale, this may indicate an abnormality of lung recoil and/or airway resistance (for example, with emphysema, pulmonary oedema, asthma or chronic lung conditions (Thelan et al 1990)). Look at the patient's position;

is the patient attempting to get into a position to aid lung expansion or particularly distressed when lying down?

2 *Sputum production* is a useful indicator of underlying lung pathology, for example, the frothy sputum associated with pulmonary oedema. Whether sputum is frothy or infected, it may be blood-stained as a result of trauma to the lung tissue. However, haemoptysis may also be due to pulmonary embolism; this would be confirmed by other symptoms (such as raised jugular venous pressure (JVP), raised temperature, pain on inspiration, tachypnoea) and the findings of a V:Q scan. If it is suspected that matter expectorated from the lungs includes stomach contents (as may occur when the oesophagus is ruptured), immediate action should be taken as the acidic nature of such aspirate can cause damage to lung tissue.

3 *Cyanosis* may be evident in two forms:
   - *central cyanosis* – occurs when large amounts of unsaturated haemoglobin are present (usually only seen when oxygen saturation has dropped to 75%);
   - *peripheral cyanosis* – indicates poor circulation.

4 *Abnormal movements* include tracheal deviation (which may indicate pneumothorax, haemothorax, massive pleural effusion or a mediastinal or lung mass) and a flail segment of the chest wall that moves inward on inspiration (paradoxical breathing), reducing tidal volume.

5 *Signs of chronic respiratory disease* include clubbing of the fingers (due to peripheral hypoxia) and a history of wheezing/shortness of breath/excessive mucus production. Patients with chronic respiratory disease also sometimes purse their lips when exhaling; this helps to keep the alveoli inflated, prolonging gas exchange.

OXYGEN SATURATION

Pulse oximetry has proved to be a major breakthrough in providing an instant, non-invasive means of assessing oxygen saturation (the carriage of oxygen on haemoglobin molecules) and has been shown to reduce the need for arterial blood gas analysis (King and Simon 1987). The amount of haemoglobin carrying oxygen (SaO_2) is expressed as a percentage of the total oxygen carrying capacity. Readings are obtained using a two-sided probe, commonly placed over the fingertip. Infrared light is passed through the fingertip; the rate of absorption varies according to the number of oxygen molecules linked to each haemoglobin molecule. Hence the pulse oximeter translates this absorption of light into a percentage reading. This reading is commonly referred to as SaO_2, although, as the reading is taken from peripheral capillaries, it is more accurately identified as SpO_2 (Woodrow 1999). The pulse oximeter also commonly displays a waveform; this reflects changes in blood flow through the capillary bed during systole and diastole. A shallow waveform displayed on the oximeter indicates poor blood flow or poor reading of the blood flow by the oximeter.

There are several situations in which pulse oximeter recordings of oxygen saturation may be unreliable, if the patient is peripherally cold the reading will be unreliable. However, it is important to be able to distinguish between readings that are unreliable because the patient is too critically ill (for example, the severely shocked patient who has peripheral vasoconstriction) and readings that are distorted through artefact affecting the signal, for example, an ill-fitting probe, nail vanish or patient movement (for example, rigors, convulsions or shivering) which will cause too much outside light to reach the sensor. The waveform displayed on the oximeter indicates the adequacy of the signal, highlighting the need for nurses to be able to recognize an abnormal waveform. Factors such as anaemia, jaundice and skin pigmentation have little or no effect on the function of the oximeter (Stoneham 1995); however, in carbon monoxide (CO) poisoning the readings will tend towards 100% as the Hb carrying the CO will register as saturated.

It is important to be aware that oxygen saturation readings can give a false sense of security for two reasons:

1 there is a potential time lag between the onset of an hypoxic event and its effects being reflected in the saturation readings (Stoneham 1995);

2 arterial oxygen saturation does not provide a picture of the overall efficiency of gas exchange, merely the transport of oxygen on the haemoglobin; the patient receiving oxygen therapy could be developing hypercapnia without showing any dramatic change in SaO_2 (Davidson and Hosie 1993).

LUNG AUSCULTATION

Listening to breath sounds is an important aspect of respiratory assessment; as airway size changes, different breath sounds are produced. These normal breath sounds are summarized in Table 4.2.

If the patient is experiencing respiratory difficulties, abnormal breath sounds may be heard. These abnormalities may include:

- *the absence of breath sounds*, for example, in pneumothorax;
- *bronchial or broncho-vesicular sounds heard over peripheral lung areas*, indicating compression/collapse of alveoli, consolidation of secretions or pleural effusion;
- *added sounds superimposed over normal or abnormal breath sounds*, such as crackles or wheezes. Crackles are caused by pressure variations in the airway and reflect the opening of collapsed alveoli or the presence of fluid in the alveoli. Wheezes are caused by narrowing or obstruction of the small airways. Wheezes can be accentuated by the administration of beta-blockers, which interfere with the broncho-dilating effects of sympathetic nervous system (SNS) stimulation.

When auscultating the patient's chest, it is essential to be familiar with normal breath sounds. As it is important to compare the two lungs the most helpful procedure is to move down the lungs fields, listening to left and right alternately. If abnormal sounds are present, it is important to identify where they are present; the larger the area of abnormal sounds, the more serious the problem. Again, knowledge of the patient's usual respiratory status is invaluable.

BLOOD GAS ANALYSIS

Concern is often expressed about the patient's oxygenation status; however, of equal if not greater importance is the level of carbon dioxide in the blood as this will affect pH. A raised carbon dioxide level causes an acidosis, affecting cellular function and (as previously discussed) the formation of oxyhaemoglobin. Acids and bases (alkalis) enter the circulation as a result of metabolism; body mechanisms that prevent these from causing an imbalance of pH are referred to as buffers.

Three buffering systems exist:

1. chemical buffers, such as bicarbonate, plasma proteins and Hb which combine with the acids/bases to reduce their effect;
2. the respiratory system which has the capacity to increase the removal of CO_2 (through hyperventilation);
3. the renal system which regulates the amount of acid and base excreted in the urine.

Arterial blood gas sampling enables analysis of the blood pH and provides the blood levels of oxygen, carbon dioxide and bicarbonate (HCO_3) (the main chemical buffer). It is used both as part of initial assessment and to evaluate the patient's response to

Table 4.2
Normal breath sounds heard on auscultation

Sound	Location	Features	Ratio of inspiration : expiration
Bronchial	Cricoid cartilage to suprasternal notch	Loud, high-pitched, hollow	1 : 2 with pause
Broncho-vesicular	Central chest ■ sternal border, intercostal spaces 1, 2 and 3 ■ between scapulae, intercostal spaces 5/6	Moderate, medium pitch, muffled	1 : 1 with pause
Vesicular	Peripheral lung areas	Soft, low pitched, rustling. Inspiration louder than expiration	5 : 2 no pause

treatment. If the patient has a suspected major chest injury, blood gas analysis should be undertaken as part of the primary survey as soon as possible after arrival in the Emergency Department (Rooney et al 2000). The normal values of arterial blood gases are provided in Table 4.3.

Normal blood pH is 7.35–7.45. An imbalance is said to occur when the pH falls (acidosis) or rises (alkalosis) outside of these parameters. In the clinical situation, much emphasis is placed on correcting an acidosis; it is important not to underestimate the significance of an alkalosis as this will decrease the offloading of oxygen at the tissues.

Generally four types of acid–base imbalance are described: metabolic or respiratory acidosis and metabolic or respiratory alkalosis. The blood gas picture for each of these is depicted in Figure 4.1.

When interpreting arterial blood gases, a step-wise approach is important:

1 Look at the pH – acidosis or alkalosis?
2 Look at the $PaCO_2$ – high, low or normal?
3 Look at the bicarbonate – high low or normal?

Table 4.4 shows an example of compensated blood gases. It is important to remember that blood gas results are never viewed in isolation but interpreted in the context of the overall condition of the patient.

THE PATIENT PRESENTING WITH BREATHLESSNESS

If the respiratory rate is greater than 20/min, it is important to determine the cause (which may be non-respiratory in origin). Be alert to possible respiratory depression, for example, from the ingestion of drugs or alcohol, or as the result of a cerebral incident.

Respiratory rate may be raised as the body is attempting to compensate for a metabolic acidosis – think about the respiratory rate of the diabetic patient admitted with ketoacidosis. It is also seen in patients with class 3 or 4 shock as the patient attempts to compensate for acidosis and hypoxia (Baskett and Nolan 2000). Other possible causes of tachypnoea are airway obstruction or constriction, infection, SNS stimulation, pain, anxiety, pyrexia or neurological problems.

Upper airway obstruction

On immediate visual assessment, the patient with upper airway obstruction is likely to have stridor; tachypnoea and/or dyspnoea; cyanosis and may be snoring. Further assessment will reveal tachycardia and lowered oxygen saturation. Blood gas analysis will show raised $PaCO_2$.

Table 4.3 Normal values for arterial blood gases		
pH	Hydrogen ion concentration	7.35–7.45
PaO_2	Partial pressure of arterial oxygen	11–13 kPa
$PaCO_2$	Partial pressure of arterial carbon dioxide	5.0–5.6 kPa
HCO_3	Bicarbonate	21–27 mmol/l

NB: Normal parameters are dependent on the reagent used. Ensure you know the norms accepted by your laboratory.

Metabolic acidosis	Metabolic alkalosis
pH falls	pH rises
$PaCO_2$ normal	$PaCO_2$ normal
HCO_3 falls	HCO_3 rises
Respiratory acidosis	Respiratory alkalosis
pH falls	pH rises
$PaCO_2$ rises	$PaCO_2$ falls
HCO_3 normal	HCO_3 normal

Figure 4.1 Types of acid–base imbalance

Table 4.4 Example of compensated blood gases	
pH	7.4
$PaCO_2$	7.0
PaO_2	8.5
HCO_3	32
SaO_2	89

The pH is normal but both the $PaCO_2$ and HCO_3 are raised. The information provided by the PaO_2 and SaO_2 indicate that this is a respiratory acidosis that has been corrected by an increase in the bicarbonate levels. It is, in fact, the blood gas picture of a patient in chronic respiratory failure.

Assessment and immediate interventions

1 Is the patient rousable?

   If not, try jaw thrust. If this relieves the symptoms (for example, obstruction, tachypnoea) put the patient into the coma position and insert an oropharyngeal or a nasopharyngeal airway if appropriate. Contact an anaesthetist and ENT surgeon (if appropriate).

2 How quickly is the patient deteriorating? Intubation, tracheostomy or cricothyroidectomy may be necessary before the anaesthetist arrives.

3 Determine the cause and intervene accordingly (see Figure 4.2).

4 Assess for patient anxiety.

   Anxiety has a profound effect on respiratory rate; aim to manage the patient in a calm and controlled environment with staff who are confident in their approach to the patient.

Remember

- Epiglottitis can occur in adults as well as children (for assessment and interventions, see Chapter 3).
- Inspiratory stridor indicates an extreme emergency – move the patient to Resus.

■ Foreign body	Remove from pharynx if possible Heimlich manoeuvre Bronchoscopy
■ Neoplasm	Helium and oxygen mixture (reduces air viscosity) Endoscopy Oro-tracheal intubation Tracheostomy
■ Epiglottitis	Helium and oxygen Lateral X-ray of neck Antibiotics Examination under anaesthetic Intubation/tracheostomy as necessary
■ Laryngospasm or anaphylaxis	Adrenaline nebulizer Intubation/tracheostomy as necessary

Figure 4.2 Interventions for airway obstruction (Singer and Webb 1994)

- A minor obstruction can suddenly deteriorate.
- Reducing patient anxiety is crucial.
- If endotracheal intubation fails, it may be necessary to proceed to cricothyroidectomy or tracheostomy. Ensure that equipment and expertise is available.
- Always consider neck trauma.

Acute dyspnoea

Assessment

- Visual assessment of respiration
- Oxygen saturation
- Lung auscultation
- Blood gas analysis
- Determine history as soon as possible (e.g. is the patient a known asthmatic?)
- Assess cardiovascular effects; start continuous ECG monitoring.

Immediate interventions

- Administer oxygen (60% via Ventimask)
- Establish venous access
- Ensure equipment and expertise is available should cardio-respiratory arrest occur.

If cardiac function is not compromised, take chest X-ray, 12-lead ECG and bloods for blood gas analysis, full blood count and urea and electrolytes.

Be alert to the following possible causes:

- Respiratory causes (e.g. asthma, respiratory alkalosis from severe hyperventilation),
- Systemic causes (e.g. metabolic acidosis, anaphylaxis, drug overdose),
- Cardiovascular causes (e.g. anaemia, left ventricular failure).

Anxiety or psychiatric causes of dyspnoea should only be considered when other possibilities have been ruled out.

Asthma

Patients with asthma are commonly hypersensitive to inhaled allergens and exhibit symptoms arising from reduced flow through the air passages. This is characteristically demonstrated by an expiratory wheeze, with air becoming trapped in the alveoli. During an acute episode, the air passages undergo a localized inflammatory response, resulting in swelling, airway constriction and bronchospasm. Asthma can also present in adults in a non-allergic form, triggered by factors such as cold weather, anxiety or exercise. An acute asthma attack is a potentially life-threatening event and must be treated accordingly.

Bronchoconstriction also occurs with severe anaphylaxis, which requires systemic treatment, hence it is important to exclude this before treating the symptoms as an acute asthmatic episode.

In life-threatening asthma, the patient will present with the following symptoms (Greaves et al 1997):

- hypotension and bradycardia;
- exhaustion and, possibly, coma;
- cyanosis, silent chest;
- peak flow < 33% of predicted.

Assessment
- Visual assessment of respiration
- Oxygen saturation
- Lung auscultation
- Blood gas analysis
- Assess for cardiovascular compromise and support accordingly
- History from relatives: onset, duration and trigger of current symptoms, past history

Immediate interventions
When anaphylaxis has been ruled out, start aggressive management (Singer and Webb 1994):

- administer high concentration O_2
- administer a beta-agonist, for example, Salbutamol via oxygen nebulizer
- administer steroids (200 mg hydrocortisone IV stat)
- IV hydration

Start continuous assessment of the following:

- ECG monitoring (heart rate/rhythm),
- SaO_2,
- BP,
- respiratory rate.

The following investigations will be required: chest X-ray; 12-lead ECG; arterial blood gases; FBC; U&Es; sputum specimen if appropriate.

Vital signs, respiratory effort and oxygen saturation are monitored to assess the patient's response to treatment. Peak expiratory flow rate should not be measured if the patient is experiencing a severe or life-threatening asthmatic episode (Kilner and Wilkinson 2000).

If the patient does not respond, the following drugs would be given successively until a response is achieved:

1 IV aminophylline with or without Ipratropium nebulizers,
2 IV salbutamol,
3 consider IV magnesium (Kaye and O'Sullivan 2002).

If the response is still inadequate, the patient may need mechanical ventilation. Antibiotics are only given in the presence of obvious infection (as indicated by fever, purulent sputum, WBC, chest X-ray).

Remember
- Fall in PaO_2 is a late sign of respiratory failure in adults.

Chest infection

Assessment
- Visual assessment of respiration
- Oxygen saturation
- Lung auscultation
- Blood gas analysis
- History: onset, duration and trigger of current symptoms, past history

Immediate interventions
- In patients without a chronic respiratory condition, oxygen therapy should be started at 0.4 FiO_2
- It is essential not to suppress cough reflex if sputum is present
- Urgently check arterial gases; chest X-ray; FBC; U&Es; blood cultures; sputum culture; viral titres
- Check whether the patient is known to the department as a patient with chronic respiratory disease and whether any advance treatment orders have been made.

> If the chest infection is not to be treated, consider sedation and analgesia
> - Ensure adequate hydration; humidify oxygen if patient is mouth breathing

1 *Bronchitis*: Bronchitis is the term given to inflamed mucosal lining of the air passages. The patient will present with symptoms of dry cough with mucoid sputum; wheeze; substernal pain. In previously healthy patients, bronchitis is usually viral requiring symptomatic treatment only.

   Patients with chronic lung disease may have bacterial or viral infection and may also present with asthmatic symptoms. History from the family is essential; the hypoxic respiratory drive will cease to function in the patient with a chronic lung condition if high levels of oxygen are administered.

2 *Pneumonia*: The patient with pneumonia will present with infective symptoms (pyrexia; tachycardia; purulent sputum). The infective process and reduced gas exchange may also be affecting the patients neurological functioning, with confusion, disorientation and aggression as possible symptoms. It may be necessary to start antibiotics immediately, however, sputum specimen and blood cultures should be collected first. It is crucial to exclude aspiration as a possible cause. Aspiration pneumonia rapidly progresses to sepsis and respiratory distress syndrome; as a consequence, the patient admitted to Emergency Department with aspiration pneumonia may already be unresponsive and may require full resuscitative measures. The antibiotics likely to be used for given forms of pneumonia are summarized in Table 4.5.

Table 4.5
Antibiotics likely to be prescribed for chest infections (Singer and Webb 1994)

Possible cause	Drug
Aspiration (for example, anaerobes)	Clindamycin Cefuroxime Metronidazole
Strep. pneumoniae *H. influenzae* *Staph. aureus*	Cefuroxime Ampicillin Flucloxacillin
Gram negative	Ceftazidime Gentamycin

Myasthenia gravis

Myasthenia gravis is an autoimmune disorder resulting from an abnormality of neurochemical transmission. Patients with myasthenia gravis have an abnormally high level of antibodies to acetylcholine, the chemical present in the synapse at the nerve motor end plate. The antibodies (anticholinesterase) result in acetylcholine being destroyed too quickly. Hence the patient will tend to experience a range of symptoms arising from the exhaustion of muscles that are in constant use:

- drooping eyelids (ptosis),
- difficulty swallowing,
- difficulty speaking,
- blurred vision,
- difficulty breathing.

> **Assessment**
> - Identify the extent of respiratory failure:
>   - visual assessment
>   - lung auscultation
>   - oxygen saturation
>   - blood gas analysis
> - Identify the extent of muscle weakness
> - Identify through history from family (and patient if possible) whether there has been any recent change in medication or activity
> - Establish whether the patient is suffering a myasthenic or cholinergic crisis
>
> **Immediate interventions**
> - Support respiratory function as appropriate; alert anaesthetist if necessary
> - Establish venous access
> - Commence drugs according to type of crisis

A patient who has myasthenia gravis may present to the Emergency Department with increasing weakness of the respiratory muscles. Vital capacity is the most useful indication of respiratory function; the patient is likely to need admission to ICU for ventilation if vital capacity is <10–15 ml/kg.

Such patients are often known to the hospital of the locality in which they live, however, given the prevalence of this in "student-age" population, all nurses working in emergency care need to be alert to the symptoms and signs of an acute exacerbation. Patients diagnosed with myasthenia are advised to wear a *MedicAlert* style bracelet or necklace. However, an undiagnosed myasthenic may be seen first at an Emergency Department.

Myasthenia Gravis is kept under control by the administration of drugs to reduce the effects of the cholinesterase. However, if the drugs are not in balance with the body's production of acetylcholine, problems arise.

Myasthenics may present to the Emergency Department with two different types of crisis:

1 *Cholinergic crisis*: Over-administration of anticholinergic drugs. The drug Edrophonium (Tensilon) may be given to diagnose cholinergic crisis (known as the Tensilon test). This is a short-acting anticholinesterase and will cause profound weakness in a patient in cholinergic crisis. Cholinergic crisis is managed using IV Atropine 1 mg given every 30 min to a maximum of 8 mg. It is essential that full resuscitative facilities are available if the Tensilon test is to be used.

2 *Myasthenic crisis*: A life-threatening episode of acute deterioration in patients diagnosed with myasthenia gravis. Anticholinergic drugs (Pyridostigmine) should be given and Azathioprine dose increased and/or steroids commenced.

It can be difficult distinguishing between the two types of crisis. However, a careful history from the patient and relatives is helpful. Most myasthenic patients are aware of impending crises and can indicate what the imbalance is.

CARDIOVASCULAR EMERGENCIES

INITIAL CARDIAC ASSESSMENT

The purpose of cardiac assessment in the Emergency Department is to enable accurate diagnosis and determine the extent of cardiovascular inadequacy.

NON-INVASIVE ASSESSMENT

1 *Pulse*: Rate and rhythm need to be observed as abnormalities of either could result in inadequate cardiac output. The site at which a pulse can be found is also a useful indicator of the patient's systolic BP (see Figure 4.3).

A palpable radial pulse indicates systolic pressure >80 mmHg
A palpable femoral pulse > 70 mmHg
A palpable carotid pulse > 60 mmHg

Figure 4.3 The relationship between palpable pulse site and systolic blood pressure

2 *Colour*: Cyanosis is an important indicator of cardiovascular function with central cyanosis characteristic of impaired gas exchange and peripheral cyanosis indicating reduced blood flow. Pallor indicates poor perfusion (as a result of catecholamine release and vasoconstriction).

3 *Capillary Refill Time*: Peripheral perfusion is best assessed using capillary refill which should be equal to or less than two seconds; any longer could indicate inadequate tissue perfusion.

4 *Skin temperature*: Skin should be assessed for localized or generalized warmth or coolness and the presence of peripheral pulses.

5 *Jugular venous pressure*: The jugular vein is usually visible when lying flat; however, when the patient is elevated to at least 45°, the vein should no longer be visible. Distended jugular veins (raised JVP) indicate either increased blood volume, vena cavae obstruction or right ventricular failure (RVF).

6 *Pain and posture*: If conscious, the patient should be asked about the site and intensity of pain, noting any guarding actions. From a cardiovascular perspective, any of these symptoms may indicate ischaemia or internal haemorrhage.

ECG MONITORING

Continuous electrocardiograph monitoring is routine practice with critically ill patients, generating information other than purely heart rate. The presence of arrhythmias may indicate electrolyte disturbance, drug toxicity (for example, Digoxin), SNS stimulation or hypoxaemia. If a patient has a pulse rate of >100 or <60 with a dysrhythmia, suspect impaired tissue perfusion.

The 12-lead ECG provides a more detailed picture of how different areas of the heart are functioning, hence enabling areas of ischaemia or infarction to be more accurately pinpointed. Positioning of the ECG leads on the four limbs enables electrical activity of the heart flowing at and between those points to

Emergency care of the adult

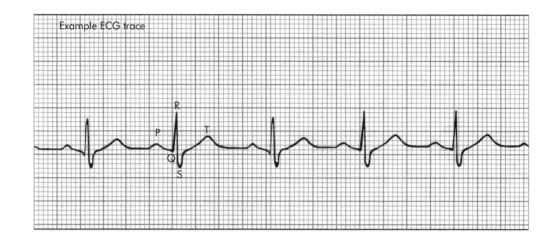

be plotted (aVR; aVL; aVF; I; II; III), whilst the more specific chest leads (V$_1$–V$_6$) plot the electrical activity at that specific point.

The following systematic approach is useful for initial analysis of the ECG waveform (after Walthall 2000):

Rhythm	Regular?
	Equal intervals between the R waves?
Rate	Sinus? (is the heartbeat originating with the P wave?)
	Tachycardia/bradycardia?
P waves	Present?
	Uniform shape?
	Do they precede the QRS complex?
QRS complex	Normal width/shape?
T waves	Are the ST segments above, on or below the isoelectric line?
	Are the T waves uniform in shape and size?
Intervals	Normals: P–R: 0.12–0.2 seconds
	QRS: 0.07–0.1 seconds
	Q–T: 0.33–0.43 seconds
	NB: P–R and Q–T intervals will vary with heart rate.

BP AND PULSE PRESSURE

Serial BP recordings can provide valuable information about blood volume, cardiac output and peripheral resistance. The difference between systolic and diastolic pressures (pulse pressure) gives a further indication of systemic vascular resistance (SVR), for example, in the hypovolaemic patient, diastolic pressure will rise initially as a result of SNS stimulation and subsequent peripheral vasoconstriction. It is important to remember that the presence of a "normal" BP does not indicate adequate tissue perfusion. When cardiac output falls, compensatory mechanisms (tachycardia, tachypnoea, peripheral vasoconstriction, decreased urine output) come into play in an attempt to maintain an adequate BP. The effects of pain and anxiety on BP must also be considered.

It is important to be aware that the use of automated devices (for example, Dinamap™) may not be effective in extremely shocked patients (Oh 1996).

CARDIAC AUSCULTATION

The normal cardiac sounds are summarized in Figure 4.4. Auscultation provides valuable additional information about the effects on the heart of the patient's current illness. S$_1$ and S$_2$ may be muffled or much louder as a result of low or raised cardiac output. During inspiration, there is a rise in venous return with prolonged right ventricular systole;

Sound	Origin
S$_1$	Closure of tricuspid and mitral valves
S$_2$	Closure of pulmonary and aortic valves
S$_3$	Rapid filling in diastole
	Normally heard only in children and young people
S$_4$	Blood rebounding on non-compliant ventricles

Figure 4.4 Normal cardiac sounds

consequently S_2 will be split with the aortic valve closing before the tricuspid. During expiration, the two valves close together, therefore a split S_2 on expiration is considered abnormal. In a patient with previously normal heart sounds, a split S_2 on expiration, could indicate left ventricular failure (LVF), pulmonary hypertension, ischaemia, myocardial infarction, right or left bundle branch block.

S_3 occurs as a result of rapid filling early in diastole, usually due to increased residual volume in the ventricles; again this can indicate RVF or LVF. S_4 is a late diastolic sound that occurs as a result of non-compliant ventricles; when the atria contract, blood bounces off the ventricular walls producing S_4. This may indicate hypertension, ventricular hypertrophy or acute myocardial infarction.

Having rapidly assimilated this information, it is important to move on to more specific observations to support initial findings (remembering that a change in observation pattern is more significant than one reading).

THE PATIENT PRESENTING WITH CHEST PAIN

Assessment
- Non-invasive assessment – airway, breathing, circulation, level of consciousness
- ECG monitoring
- BP
- Oxygen saturation
- Assess nature and site of pain – rapidly identify whether it is cardiac in origin
- Chest X-ray

Immediate interventions
- Need for pain relief and anti-emetic as soon as possible
- Establish venous access
- High flow, high concentration FiO_2 unless known to have chronic respiratory problem

Pain relief should be given as soon as possible, that is, when you have information about the probable cause. The goal should be to give optimum analgesia (neither excessive or insufficient). Insufficient pain relief will result in reduced respiratory effort, whilst excessive analgesia may mask important symptoms.

P	Palliative/provocative – what relieves/exacerbates the pain; what triggered this episode?
Q	Quality of pain – burning, sharp, stabbing
R	Region and radiation of the pain
S	Severity – rating the pain (verbally) on a score of 0 (none) to 10 (most severe) can be helpful
T	Temporal – when did/does it start and how long does it last?

Figure 4.5 The PQRST mnemonic for assessing chest pain

Table 4.6
Types of chest pain and possible causes (Singer and Webb 1994)

Type of pain	Possible cause
Sharp pain exacerbated by breathing	Pleuritic (infection or embolus) Musculo-skeletal Pericardial
Dull continuous pressing pain	Myocardial ischaemia or infarction Pneumothorax
Tender to touch	Musculo-skeletal (for example, costochondritis; myalgia; trauma)
Pain related to body position	Reflux oesophagitis Pericarditis
Sharp pain or ache related to meals	Peptic, occasionally cardiac

In order to assess chest pain, the PQRST mnemonic can be useful (see Figure 4.5).

The type of pain that the patient reports gives an early indication of the possible underlying cause (see Table 4.6), although it must be remembered that some of the terms used to describe pain are subjective. Hence the type of pain reported by the patient should not be taken in isolation from other symptoms.

Angina

Angina results from inadequate oxygen delivery to the cardiac tissue, usually caused by narrowing of the coronary arteries. The patient with angina will commonly report central chest pain that may radiate to the jaw and arms. The onset of angina indicates either additional demand for oxygen (possibly due to exertion or anxiety) or a reduced supply of oxygen (due to further narrowing of the coronary arteries, or through systemic hypoxia caused by respiratory problems). It is safer to assume that the patient with angina has suffered a myocardial infarction until cardiac enzyme and ECG results contradict this diagnosis. If angina is occurring with increasing frequency and after little exertion, the patient is likely to be admitted for review of his current therapy.

In patients with cardiac pain, the 12-lead ECG is key to identifying which area of the heart is suffering from ischaemic damage, and whether the patient has suffered a myocardial infarction.

Assessment
- Non-invasive assessment – airway, breathing, circulation, level of consciousness
- continuous ECG monitoring and 12-lead ECG
- BP
- Oxygen saturation
- Assess nature and site of pain

Immediate interventions
- Total rest
- Establish venous access
- Treat pain (e.g. IV Nitrates)
- Manage arrhythmias
  – Calcium antagonist
  – Beta-blocker if not contraindicated (asthma, vascular disease, cardiac disease)
- Anticoagulant therapy (aspirin and IV Heparin)
- Inform cardiologist

It is important to monitor cardiovascular response to drugs, particularly those with vasodilating action (see Table 4.7), to ensure that BP does not drop too quickly. The patient should also be warned to expect flushing, warmth in the limbs and headache as side effects of vasodilation. A reduction in pain indicates success of the initial drug therapy. However, the patient is likely to be admitted if changes are seen on the ECG. The patient's previous hospital records are crucial in this decision-making process (and increasingly easy to access electronically). If the patient is to be discharged, it is essential to check their understanding of current medication and lifestyle, particularly if over-exertion has contributed to their latest episode of angina.

Table 4.7
Cardiovascular drugs categorized according to therapeutic goal

Goal	Category of drug
Reduce circulating volume (preload)	Diuretics (particularly loop diuretics such as frusemide); nitrates
Increase contraction of cardiac muscle	Inotropes (for example, dopamine; dobutamine)
Reduce peripheral resistance (afterload)	Vasodilators: beta-blockers; calcium channel blockers (diltiazem); nitrates; ACE inhibitors (captopril; enalopril)
Increase blood flow through coronary arteries	Nitrates; calcium antagonists

Myocardial infarction

The patient presenting with a diagnosis of suspected myocardial infarction tends to have symptoms of cardiac insufficiency, due to reduced ventricular activity. Hence the patient will have some or all of the following symptoms:

- lowered BP,
- tachycardia (or bradycardia with an inferior infarction),
- tachypnoea or dyspnoea,
- a degree of peripheral shutdown (cold and clammy),
- pulmonary oedema.

Immediate goals are to

1 confirm diagnosis of myocardial infarction,
2 reperfuse injured tissue where possible,
3 prevent further damage to ischaemic tissue,
4 identify and correct arrhythmias and cardiac failure arising from the loss of blood supply to infarcted myocardial cells.

Diagnosis is confirmed through raised levels of cardiac enzymes (released when myocardial cells are damaged) and changes in the pattern of electrical activity, as seen on a 12-lead ECG and via continuous monitoring. Chest X-ray may also be indicated if pulmonary oedema (LVF) is suspected.

Ruth Endacott

Table 4.8
Absolute and relative contraindications to thrombolysis

Absolute contraindications	Relative contraindications
■ Serious trauma or major surgery within past month ■ Active GI bleeding ■ Aortic aneurysm ■ Cerebral surgery or injury within past 2 months ■ Cerebral neoplasm or aneurysm ■ Diastolic B/P > 100 mmHg	■ Prior organ biopsy within past month ■ Proliferative diabetic retinopathy ■ Bleeding diathesis (e.g. major vessel rupture) if not compressible ■ Prolonged or traumatic CPR ■ Recent obstetric delivery

Assessment

■ Non-invasive assessment – airway, breathing, circulation, level of consciousness
■ ECG monitoring and 12-lead ECG
■ BP – be alert for cardiogenic shock
■ Oxygen saturation
■ Assess nature and site of pain

Immediate interventions

■ Accurate diagnosis
■ Secure venous access
■ Initiate thrombolysis if appropriate
■ Oxygen therapy
■ Pain control with anti-emetic
■ Give anti-arrhythmic drugs as appropriate
■ Insertion of a CVP line if worsening LVF

Thrombolysis should be given as soon as possible after the onset of symptoms and ideally within 12 hours but may be effective for up to 18–24 hours after onset of symptoms (if pain is still present). Abnormal electrical activity results from both infarcted and injured/ ischaemic areas of myocardium, hence reperfusing injured and ischaemic tissues will result in some of the electrical activity returning to normal. In particular, ST elevation will disappear. Revascularization arrhythmias are common and largely transient but should be monitored.

A key nursing role when thrombolytic drugs are to be administered lies in identifying possible contraindications, from other symptoms and signs (see Table 4.8). Some contraindications are absolute; other, less serious, contraindications have to be weighed against the benefits of giving the thromobolytic drug. Absolute and relative contraindications may vary between medications and may be influenced by local policy; they may also change as new evidence emerges.

If the area of infarcted myocardium is in the left ventricle, LVF, and pulmonary oedema, will result. This can be sudden and severe and may progress quickly to cardiogenic shock, with possible hypoxic damage to other organs (for example, brain and kidneys). In order to effectively and speedily manage LVF and cardiogenic shock, a CVP line will be inserted. This enables titration of drugs against overall circulating volume. The pulmonary oedema seen in myocardial infarction patients results from the inability of the left ventricle to empty effectively, causing backlog in the pulmonary circulation, with fluid passing from pulmonary capillaries into the alveoli. This reduces the surface area available for gas exchange in the alveoli and results in hypoxia. Consequently, the blood that is pumped from the left ventricle is not only inadequate in volume but carrying less oxygen (see Figure 4.6) leading rapidly to cardiogenic shock if unchecked.

Pulmonary embolism

Pulmonary embolism commonly occurs secondary to deep vein thrombosis (which may or may not have been diagnosed). A part of the thrombus breaks off to form an embolus and moves along the venous circulation to the pulmonary circulation where it blocks a pulmonary capillary, causing infarction to the lung tissue supplied by that capillary. The extent of the damage, and symptoms seen when the patient presents at the Emergency Department, depends on the size of the embolus and, therefore, where it lodges in the pulmonary circulation. Diagnosis is confirmed by a V:Q (ventilation:perfusion) scan of the lungs. The patient may present with multiple emboli, arising from a thrombus fragmenting and blocking several, usually small, areas of lung tissue.

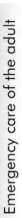

Emergency care of the adult

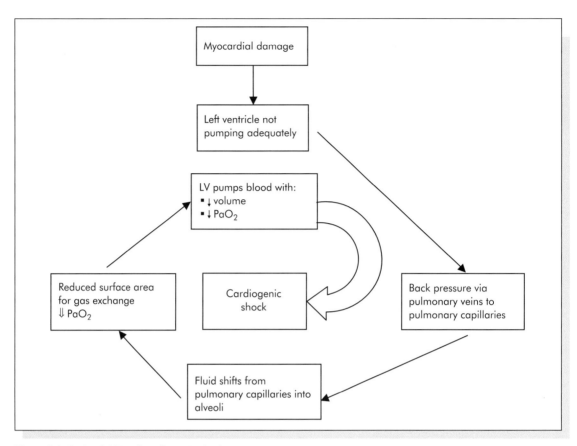

Figure 4.6 Cycle of LVF and cardiogenic shock

As highlighted in Table 4.1, effective gas exchange and tissue oxygenation are dependent on adequate pulmonary circulation. Hence the patient with pulmonary embolism may present with hypoxic consequences as severe as

- loss of consciousness,
- cyanosis,
- tachycardia,
- hypotension,
- dyspnoea.

Even with a small embolism, the patient will show signs of fatigue and dyspnoea, although it is easy to confuse these signs with other respiratory problems. Haemoptysis may be present.

Pulmonary embolism can also be caused by air, fat or amniotic fluid emboli. These are less common but cause the same effects.

Assessment
- Visual assessment of respiratory function
- ECG monitoring and 12-lead ECG
- BP
- Oxygen saturation and arterial blood gas analysis
- Lung auscultation
- Assess nature and site of pain
- Blood for clotting screen
- V:Q scan (Ventilation:Perfusion)

Immediate interventions
- High concentration oxygen therapy
- Secure venous access
- Administer anticoagulants
- Monitor cardiac rhythm

Aortic aneurysm

An aneurysm is an abnormality or weakness of the wall of an artery, commonly the aorta, resulting in bulging or splitting of the inner lining (the latter referred to as a dissecting aneurysm). Once the artery wall has weakened in this manner, it can leak or, more fatally, rupture. The patient will present with symptoms of hypovolaemia:

- hypotension,
- peripheral shutdown,
- pallor,
- tachypnoea,
- lower limbs may show reduced perfusion and increased capillary refill time.

The aneurysm if in the descending aorta in the abdomen can usually be palpated or occasionally present a visible palpating abdominal mass. If it is suspected that the patient has a dissecting thoracic aortic aneurysm, blood pressure should be checked in both arms.

The patient will need urgent surgery and correction of hypovolaemia, with blood and colloid fluid.

Assessment
- Non-invasive assessment – airway, breathing, circulation, level of consciousness
- ECG monitoring
- BP
- Oxygen saturation
- Assess nature and site of pain
- Abdominal ultrasound may be performed

Immediate interventions
- Oxygen therapy
- Secure venous access
- Fluid replacement titrated to BP
- Analgesia
- Prepare patient and family for surgery

NEUROLOGICAL EMERGENCIES

INITIAL NEUROLOGICAL ASSESSMENT

There are three main causes of neurological brain dysfunction:

1 interruption in oxygen delivery to brain cells (for example, reduced blood supply or reduced oxygenation – respiratory disease; reduced body temperature);
2 change in cell chemistry, for example, metabolic – hypo/hyperglycaemia; renal failure; hypercalcaemia; myxoedema; poisoning; encephalopathy;
3 damage to or pressure on the brain cells (not hypoxic), for example, tumour; meningitis; haemorrhage.

If you suspect that a patient may have a neurological problem affecting brain function, undertake the assessment with these three in mind. However, as the brain is also the "conductor" of other organs, neurological assessment is always carried out in conjunction with respiratory and cardiac assessment. Similarly, neurological problems that the patient presents with at the Emergency Department may be the result of underlying disease of another body system, for example, the respiratory, cardiovascular or hepatic system. Until you have established the cause, assume that the patient's vital functions may deteriorate.

Neurological functioning must also be assessed in relation to the rest of the nervous system:

- motor nerve function,
- sensory nerve function.

It is essential that this assessment is set against the patient's normal functioning in order to distinguish between the acute presenting problem and any pre-existing neurological condition (for example, multiple sclerosis or Parkinson's Disease).

A clear history is essential in identifying the cause of the presenting problems, for example:

1 Has the change in level of consciousness or nerve function been progressive or sudden?
2 Has the patient been confused or aggressive of late?
3 Has the patient experienced any tremors?

Assessment of consciousness can be undertaken using the AVPU tool (see Figure 4.7).

Consistency in recording of neurological assessment is crucial; the pattern of patient response over a few recordings (see Figure 4.8) will determine the speed and nature of interventions required.

A more detailed picture of neurological functioning is obtained using the Glasgow Coma Score (GCS – see Figure 4.9). Scores in each of the three categories are commonly added to give an overall GCS score. This information is frequently used by pre-hospital

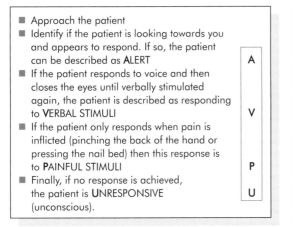

- ■ Approach the patient
- ■ Identify if the patient is looking towards you and appears to respond. If so, the patient can be described as ALERT
- ■ If the patient responds to voice and then closes the eyes until verbally stimulated again, the patient is described as responding to VERBAL STIMULI
- ■ If the patient only responds when pain is inflicted (pinching the back of the hand or pressing the nail bed) then this response is to PAINFUL STIMULI
- ■ Finally, if no response is achieved, the patient is UNRESPONSIVE (unconscious).

A

V

P

U

Figure 4.7 AVPU tool for assessing level of consciousness

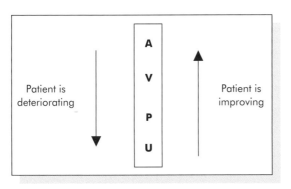

Patient is deteriorating

A
V
P
U

Patient is improving

Figure 4.8 Use of AVPU over time to indicate patient progress

Eyes open	Spontaneously	4
	To speech	3
	To pain	2
	None	1
Best verbal response	Orientated	5
	Confused	4
	Inappropriate words	3
	Incomprehensible sounds	2
	None	1
Best motor response	Obey commands	6
	Localise pain	5
	Withdraws from pain (normal flexion)	4
	Abnormal flexion to pain	3
	Extension to pain	2
	None	1

Figure 4.9 The Glasgow Coma Score

Table 4.9
Patterns of vital signs relating to neurological problems

BP	Pulse	Respiratory rate	Temperature
Raised ICP			
High systolic BP Wide pulse pressure	Slow	Abnormal rate or rhythm	May elevate
High spinal cord injury			
Low	Slow	May be slow	Low
Brain stem injury			
Fluctuates	Fluctuates	Abnormal rate or rhythm	May elevate

care providers to communicate an overall picture of the patients condition and any change during transport to the Emergency Department.

This is used with other key vital signs (pulse, BP, respiratory rate, temperature) plus pupil reaction and limb movements to determine the patient's overall condition. This combination of vital signs also provides an indicator of the likely site of any neurological problems (see Table 4.9).

MANAGING THE PATIENT WITH IMPAIRED CONSCIOUSNESS

Assessment
Airway, breathing, circulation
GCS
AVPU
Vital signs
History from relatives: onset, duration and trigger of current symptoms, past history

Immediate interventions
Overall priorities with the unresponsive patient are

1 to preserve or restore function of vital organs,
2 to prevent further damage to vital organs,
3 to determine cause.

Immediate interventions are shown in Figure 4.10.

Ruth Endacott

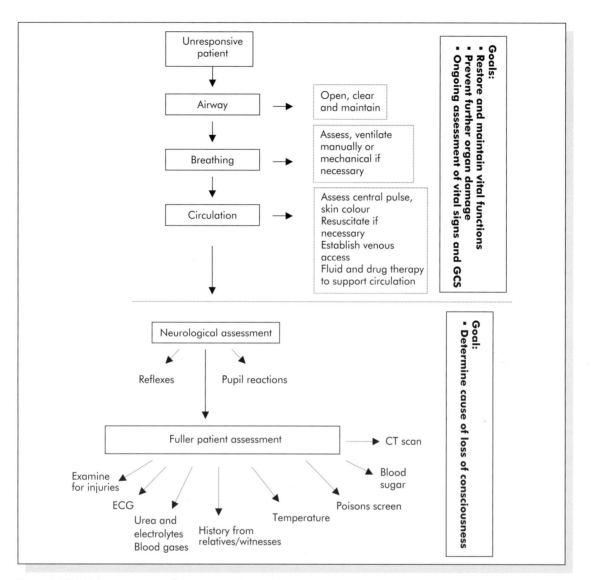

Figure 4.10 Initial management of the unresponsive patient

Meningitis

Whilst most commonly seen in children, meningitis does also present in the adult population. Rapid detection is essential, particularly with the more virulent meningococcal form. Sources of infection for meningitis are varied, and may arise from within the spinal column or the systemic circulation. Alternatively, infection may enter the cerebro-spinal fluid from trauma to the skull, eroding neoplasms or septic foci in the brain tissue.

Symptoms tend to be progressive and may start with something as minor as flu-like symptoms, commencing with headache and neckache and descending to the back and legs. The severity of pain may result in overt crying in adults (Adam and Osborne 1997), and nausea, vomiting, fever and photophobia are frequently seen. Irritability can progress to drowsiness and fitting, and the patient may rapidly become unresponsive. A positive Kernig's sign may or may not be present (extension of one knee with hip fully flexed produces pain and spasm in the hamstrings).

Meningococcal meningitis is usually accompanied by a distinctive rash.

Management of meningitis focuses on monitoring and controlling the symptoms and precise diagnosis to guide antibiotic therapy. Investigations include CT scan, lumbar punctures, blood and CSF cultures. Neurological assessment is key to identifying further deterioration, particularly where trends are developing. Symptom control is attempted using cooling measures (for example, fan therapy and antipyretic drugs); analgesia and minimal handling. Antibiotic administration may initially be guided by clinical assessment, prior to microbiology results. Steroid administration has not been shown to be of benefit in the adult population.

Non-traumatic cerebral bleed/clot

The presentation and management of the patient with a cerebral bleed will depend on the likely location, as shown in Table 4.10.

Other vascular problems include brainstem haematoma and development of aneurysms. The brainstem haematoma can be caused by primary injury (direct causes) or secondary insults of hypoxia, or increased intracranial pressure. The main clinical signs are

- rapid progression of fluctuating vital signs,
- decerebrate posturing,
- bilateral pathological posturing.

An aneurysm is a localized dilation or sac that develops due to congenital or acquired factors. Maldevelopment of the middle muscular vessel layer (media) is an important factor; a concurrent weakness of the internal muscular vessel layer (intima) is also an enhancing factor. There are five general types of aneurysm:

1 *Berry/saccular* – congenital, developmental at the bifurcations, usually in the Circle of Willis. Common sites include the posterior communicating, internal carotid, anterior cerebral or middle cerebral vessel areas. These are usually small, <15 mm and appear berry-like with a stem or neck.
2 *Fusiform/giant* – caused by hypertension, atherosclerosis. These are more common in the basilar and carotid arteries. The appearance is a large vessel dilation, usually 3–5 cm in size and often

with a twisted appearance. It will act as a space-occupying lesion, and is less likely to rupture.
3 *Mycotic/septic emboli* – are a rare form, usually located in smaller/terminal vessels, and tend to occur in multiple sites concurrently. The septic emboli erode the layers of the arterial wall (erosive vasculitis).
4 *Charcot–Bouchard* – are caused by chronic hypertension, microscopic in size, and also occur in multiples. These are usually located in the basal ganglia and brainstem.

Aneurysms can also occur due to traumatic or shearing forces.

The signs and symptoms are defined by pre-rupture, and during/post-rupture phases:

- *Pre-rupture* is mostly asymptomatic:
  – enlargement: headache, extra ocular muscle changes (CN III, IV, VI palsy), diplopia, blurred vision;
  – leakage – headache, nausea, neck/back pain, malaise, photophobia.
- *During/post-rupture* – more symptomatic – includes headache, alteration in level of consciousness, dizziness, vomiting, cranial nerve dysfunction, and visual changes. Signs of meningeal irritation include – photophobia, irritability, and positive Kernig's Sign.

Diagnostic investigations include CT and MRI scans, cerebral angiography and lumbar puncture. Management includes bed rest with head of bed elevation; sedation; maintenance of a dark environment; control of hypertension; avoidance of vagal stimulation and surgical clipping if appropriate (for example, Berry aneurysm). The main complications are re-bleeding, especially on days 7–10, vasospasm, increased intracranial pressure and hydrocephalus.

ENDOCRINE EMERGENCIES
Diabetic ketoacidosis

The diabetic patient presenting at the Emergency Department is likely to have changes in level of consciousness. Prompt assessment of blood sugar levels will determine whether the problem is hypo or hyper glycaemic. Whilst both are potentially life threatening, the ketoacidosis that accompanies

Ruth Endacott

Table 4.10
Recognizing and managing cerebral haemorrhage

Causes	Clinical presentation	Management
Subarachnoid haemorrhage (A bleed between the arachnoid and pia mater layers, collecting in the subarachnoid space)		
Fall	*Grade 1: minimal* – asymptomatic, alert, minimal headache, no neuro deficits	Diagnosis includes CAT scan. Treatment is also based on surgical evacuation of the haematoma and control of haemorrhage.
Anatomical defect	*Grade 2: mild* – alert, mild to severe headache, minimal neuro deficit (central nervous/cranial nerve dysfunction)	Complications include increased ICP, clot recummulation, delayed haemorrhage and seizures
	Grade 3: moderate – drowsy, confused, may have focal deficits	
	Grade 4: moderate to severe – stupor, mild to severe hemiparesis, possible early decerebration	
	Grade 5: severe – deep coma, decerebration, moribund appearance	
	Concurrent symptoms also include photophobia, headache, projectile vomiting, seizures and blood stained CSF	
Intracerebral haematoma (A well-defined blood clot deep in the brain tissue or parenchyma)		
Non-traumatic causes	Dependent on size and location. Level of consciousness may deteriorate and progress to coma	Goal is to allow reabsorption to occur. Frontal or temporal lobe haematomas have a 90% mortality
Overdose of cocaine, crack or amphetamines	Increased mortality with co-existent DIC, hypoxia, hypotension and alcohol abuse	

hyperglycaemia makes this a more complex situation to manage. Inability of the body to utilize the circulating glucose results in fat metabolism, with resultant release of ketones and metabolic acidosis.

Assessment
- Airway, breathing, circulation
- GCS/AVPU
- Blood sugar (fingertip and laboratory analysis)
- Vital signs
- Fluid balance
- Blood gas analysis
- History from patient and/or relatives: onset, duration and trigger of current symptoms, past history.

Immediate interventions
- Rapid assessment of impact on other organs (through reduced perfusion and acidosis)
- Rapid assessment of electrolyte and acid–base status
- Commence insulin infusion
- The patient does not have to be comatose for the condition to be life threatening; the major problem with hyperglycaemia is the resultant electrolyte and acid–base imbalance
- Look for the trigger for the hyperglycaemia – possibly an MI or sepsis
- The overall aim is *gradual* replacement of fluids and gradual reduction of glucose levels.

There can be severe fluid loss with diabetic keto-acidosis; however, the type of fluid used needs to be matched to the patient's electrolyte status. Blood should be sent for urgent U&Es analysis.

The patient may also have hypovolaemic shock due to excessive fluid loss hence it is important to restore circulating blood volume with colloid solutions. It *may* be necessary to insert a CVP line for more accurate assessment of fluid status. However, fluid replacement should be undertaken gradually to avoid cardiac failure as the underlying cause of the crisis may be a cardiac event. Infusion of insulin causes shift of potassium into the cells, hence potassium may need to be added to intravenous fluids, according to the patient's electrolyte status.

A nasogastric tube should be placed if the patient's level of consciousness is impaired, to counter the risk of aspiration from delayed gastric emptying.

Hypoglycaemia

Assessment
- Airway, breathing, circulation
- GCS/AVPU
- Vital signs
- Assess hydration
- History from patient and/or relatives: onset, duration and trigger of current symptoms, past history

Immediate interventions
- Oral glucose if conscious
- IV glucose and/or glucagon if unconscious
- Protect airway if necessary

The symptoms of hypoglycaemia include:

- altered level of consciousness or seizures,
- nausea and/or vomiting,
- sweating and tachycardia.

If the patient is conscious, give oral glucose. In addition, carbohydrate should be given (for example, in sandwiches) to provide longer term glucose replacement. If the patient is unconscious, venous access should be obtained and glucose given IV (25–50 ml 50% glucose as a bolus). If venous access is not available, give glucose via nasogastric tube or give glucagon I/M or SC. Glucagon will stimulate the conversion of glycogen back to glucose, raising the blood sugar level.

Consider the underlying cause:

- organ disease (liver, adrenal glands or pituitary gland),
- over-medication with insulin or sulphonamides,
- inadequate food intake,
- systemic infection,
- excess alcohol intake or quinine therapy.

If the hypoglycaemia is secondary to long-acting sulphonylureas (oral antidiabetic tablet), the patient will have to be admitted for review of drug therapy. If the patient is to be discharged, check understanding of the patient and family regarding the management of diabetes.

The patient presenting with seizures

Assessment
- Airway, breathing, circulation
- GCS
- AVPU
- Vital signs, including temperature
- History from patient and/or relatives: onset, duration and trigger of current symptoms, past history

Immediate interventions
- If seizures are prolonged, it is important to bring them under control to prevent further hypoxaemic cerebral damage, reduce cerebral oxygen requirement and reduce ICP
- Recovery position
- High flow oxygen
- Administer drug therapy as appropriate (see Table 4.11)

The majority of seizures are self-limiting, hence no more needs to be done than to protect the patient from harming himself. If the patient is a known epileptic, check anticonvulsant levels.

If seizures do not respond to drug therapy, it may be necessary to intubate and ventilate the patient, in order to administer drugs which would have respiratory depressant side effects. It is important to monitor temperature; hyperthermia can occur with on-going seizures, with potential for cerebral damage.

Drugs overdose and poisons

Managing the patient following drug overdose from attempted suicide brings with it a raft of legal and ethical problems, not least whether the patient is consenting to treatment. Where the patient is unresponsive, the emergency team can take action on the basis of the life-threatening nature of the situation. However, the conscious patient may sue for assault if treatment is given without consent. It is important to note that attempting suicide does not automatically mean the patient falls within the remit of the 1983 Mental Health Act. Castledine (1994) argues that an irrational decision can still be a (legally) competent decision. It is important that these issues are discussed fully and approaches agreed amongst the Emergency Department team before such a situation arises.

Table 4.11
Drugs commonly administered during seizures (Singer and Webb 1994)

Benzodiazepines	Causes respiratory depression and hypoxaemia Ensure patient is monitored
Chlormethiazole	Causes respiratory depression and hypoxaemia Ensure patient is monitored Is an "electrolyte-free" solution so may cause electrolyte imbalances if given in large doses
Phenytoin	Should not be given intravenously if the patient is on oral dose and levels are not known Monitor ECG when giving phenytoin
Thiamine	Can also be given to known alcoholics
Magnesium sulphate	Can be useful for unremitting seizures

Patients may also be admitted with accidental drug overdose following recreational drug use, or following accidental ingestion of a poisonous substance. In any of these situations, information must be sought from those accompanying the patient or from the patient himself (see Figure 4.11).

Assessment
- Airway, breathing, circulation
- GCS/AVPU
- Vital signs, particularly temperature
- History from relatives: onset, duration and trigger of current symptoms, past history (see Figure 4.11)
- Blood screen for poisons; clotting; U&Es;

Immediate interventions
- Assess vital functions and commence resuscitative measures as necessary
- Protect airway if necessary
- Ascertain history/establish likely agent involved
- Administer antidote if appropriate

- Instigate cooling measures if appropriate – rapid diuresis if the patient is overloaded and replacement with cooled fluids
- Manage seizures with artificial ventilation, sedation and paralysis if necessary

Drugs such as ecstasy (MDMA) cause hyperpyrexia, which may go unnoticed when the drug is taken in a rave or nightclub setting. This will add to the thirst induced by the drug and result in excessive fluid intake. Coupled with the advice given to intentional users of MDMA to "drink plenty of water", the extreme picture which can develop is one of excess fluid overload (MDMA is also an anti-diuretic drug), leading to cerebral oedema and sudden collapse. The patient can rapidly proceed to multisystem failure.

Drugs which cause CNS stimulation (for example, amphetamines) can also cause hypertension which may lead to haemorrhage, commonly intracranial.

Treatment of drug overdose is therefore largely symptomatic. However, it should be remembered that drugs such as MDMA are commonly taken with other recreational drugs, hence the clinical picture is likely to be complicated (Williams et al 1998).

- **What was ingested?** Was anyone present at the time to verify the history? Are there any empty or partially filled drug containers at home or at the scene?
- **How much was taken?** If drug containers are available, calculate the missing tablets from the initial amount prescribed, taking into account the date on the prescription.
- **When were the drugs taken?** Take into account the time the person was last seen and the time when symptoms of intoxication began if the timing is not clear.
- **What was the route of administration?** Was the drug swallowed; injected (IV, IM OR SC); smoked; inhaled or snorted?
- **Does the patient have a history of substance misuse, depression or schizophrenia?**
- **What is the patient medical history?** Past and present prescription drugs; allergies; recent hospital admissions or GP attendances.

Figure 4.11 Information to be sought regarding a patient who has taken a drug overdose (after Holt 2000)

HEAT ILLNESS/INJURY
Hypothermia

A patient is said to be hypothermic if the core temperature is below 35°C. As the body's metabolic processes slow dramatically with cooling, it is impossible to assess the patient properly whilst he is still hypothermic. Hence re-warming and support of vital functions are a priority. Metabolic acidosis is common due to reduced tissue perfusion. Physiological effects of hypothermia are presented in Figure 4.12.

Assessment
- Airway, breathing, circulation
- GCS/AVPU
- Vital signs
- ECG monitoring and 12-lead ECG
- Blood gas analysis
- Blood sugar (fingertip and laboratory analysis)
- Blood screen for FBC; clotting; U&Es
- History from relatives: onset, duration and trigger of current symptoms, past history

Immediate interventions
- Check for palpable pulses; if absent, proceed to resuscitation
- Active or passive re-warming as appropriate
- Treatment of cardiac arrhythmias

Further investigations will be needed to determine the underlying cause where this is not obvious (for example, a near-drowning incident); other possible causes might be: cerebral incident; hypoglycaemia; poisoning; exposure; hypopituitarism; hypothyroidism; sepsis.

During cardiac arrest, CPR must continue until the patient is normothermic. This can mean undertaking CPR for a period of some hours. Re-warming methods used depend on the extent of the hypothermia:

- <28°C – active re-warming: surface (heated blanket) and central (gastric, peritoneal and/or bladder lavage);
- 29–33°C – surface re-warming (hypothermia blanket).

During re-warming, be aware of the following:

- Core temperature may fall as cold blood from peripheral circulation returns to the central circulation.

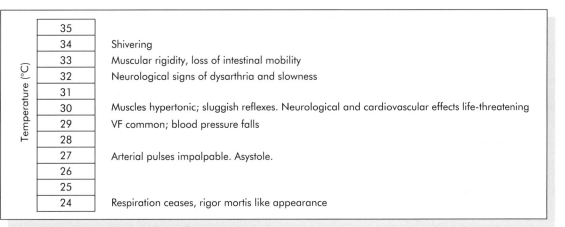

Temperature (°C)	
35	
34	Shivering
33	Muscular rigidity, loss of intestinal mobility
32	Neurological signs of dysarthria and slowness
31	
30	Muscles hypertonic; sluggish reflexes. Neurological and cardiovascular effects life-threatening
29	VF common; blood pressure falls
28	
27	Arterial pulses impalpable. Asystole.
26	
25	
24	Respiration ceases, rigor mortis like appearance

Figure 4.12 Physiological effects of hypothermia

Table 4.12 Physiological effects of hyperthermia by system	
Respiratory effects	Tachypnoea Respiratory alkalosis
Cardiovascular effects	Tachycardia ECG changes (ST depression and T wave flattened) Cardiac failure (late sign)
Nervous system effects	Confusion, delirium, convulsions, papillary abnormalities, coma
Fluid and electrolyte balance	Loss of fluid, sodium potassium, calcium and magnesium from excessive sweating
Renal effects	Acute renal failure Rhabdomyolysis (later)

- As tissues are re-perfused during re-warming, metabolic acidosis can worsen.
- Hypovolaemia will worsen as peripheral circulation re-opens.
- Arrhythmias may occur.

Hyperthermia

Hyperthermia is said to occur when the core temperature rises above 41°C. The patient will show signs of delirium with a core temperature between 40°C and

Assessment
- Airway, breathing, circulation
- GCS/AVPU
- Vital signs
- ECG monitoring and 12-lead ECG
- Blood for U&Es; clotting; drugs screen (if appropriate)
- History from relatives: onset, duration and trigger of current symptoms, past history

Immediate interventions
- Maximum FiO_2
- Active cooling until temperature reduces to <39°C:
  - Remove clothing
  - Cool environment
  - Surface cooling (fan, tepid sponge)
- May be drug-induced – ecstasy; alcohol; phenothiazines; butyrophenones – hence consider other effects of those drugs.

42°C and coma above 42–43°C. The most severe effects of hyperthermia are on the nervous system; however, other effects will be seen (see Table 4.12).

Active cooling will focus on surface interventions; however, internal cooling may also be indicated (gastric lavage; bladder lavage; peritoneal lavage). Patient may also require urgent ventilation to allow paralysis (to prevent shivering). It is important to minimize handling of the patient where possible.

ABDOMINAL PAIN

Assessment
- Vital signs – airway, breathing, circulation
- Urgent exclusion of dissecting or leaking aortic aneurysm
- Observe vomit/stools for blood, mucus
- History from relatives: onset, duration and trigger of current symptoms, past history
- Exclude pregnancy in women of child-bearing age
- Pain assessment: character, duration, frequency, location, distribution and aggravating/relieving factors

Immediate interventions
- Send stool/vomit specimen for analysis
- Fluid replacement if hypovolaemic

Possible causes of abdominal pain:

- mucosal irritation;
- muscle spasm (for example, biliary colic, renal colic, entero-colitis);
- capsular stretching (enlarged liver or spleen);
- peritoneal inflammation;
- referred medical cause, for example, diabetes or MI.

Severe vomiting may indicate a central nervous system problem (for example, Menieres disease); paralytic ileus; delayed gastric emptying; metabolic causes; drug induced (including chemotherapy).

History of stools/bowel movements – recent blood, mucous or diarrhoea. If the patient has severe diarrhoea also take a history of recent travel.

Perforation/obstruction

Obstruction of the bowel should always be considered a potentially life-threatening event and may lead to perforation and peritonitis. The three goals of emergency management of the patient are to

1 assess the nature and extent of bowel dysfunction,
2 assess and support the function of other organs,
3 relieve pressure within the abdomen if possible.

The bowel can become obstructed due to interruption of the blood supply (for example, mesenteric embolus); interruption of the nerve supply (for example, paralytic ileus) or twisting of the bowel (for example, volvulus, or hernia). If the bowel stops working, there will be a collection of fluid, gas and faeces above the obstruction and consequent swelling of the bowel. As the bowel swells, blood supply to the bowel wall will become obstructed and the bowel will become ischaemic or infarcted. A severe metabolic acidosis will develop. The site of the obstruction can be determined by the nature, site and intensity of pain, and the nature of vomit. Faecal fluid will sometimes be vomited when the patient has a large bowel obstruction.

Assessment
- Vital signs – look for signs of hypovolaemic shock or peritonitis
- Blood gases
- Blood for FBC; U&Es; pancreatic amylase
- Abdominal X-ray
- History from relatives: onset, duration and trigger of current symptoms, past history
- Pain assessment

Immediate interventions
- Oxygen therapy
- Establish venous access
- IV fluid to correct hypovolaemia
- Analgesia
- Nil orally
- Insert a nasogastric tube to drain the upper gastro-intestinal tract
- Prepare the patient for the possibility of surgery

Prophylactic antibiotics are likely to be prescribed to reduce the risk of peritonitis should the bowel perforate. Peritonitis should be suspected if the patient describes wide-spread pain across the abdomen, with a reluctance to move or allow palpation. The abdomen is usually distended and rigid and the patient's respirations will be shallow, due to both the abdominal distension and severe abdominal pain on deep inspiration.

Appendicitis

A diagnosis of appendicitis is commonly made according to the pattern of pain described by the patient. Pain from appendicitis is commonly felt as a dull ache

Ruth Endacott

originating in the mid abdomen and spreading to the right lower quadrant (RLQ) of the abdomen. The general diagnostic pattern is one of referred pain; pain is felt in the RLQ when the left lower quadrant (LLQ) is palpated; pain is felt in the left upper abdomen when McBurney's point (2 in. from the iliac crest in line with the umbilicus) is palpated. The patient is often vomiting and may have diarrhoea. More generalized abdominal pain in addition to this specific pattern may indicate perforation and peritonitis.

Assessment
- Vital signs
- History from relatives: onset, duration and trigger of current symptoms, past history
- Pain assessment
- Observe for signs of peritonitis
- Bloods for FBC; U&Es; glucose

Immediate interventions
- Nil orally
- Establish venous access
- Intravenous fluids if dehydrated
- Analgesia
- Prepare for surgery

Gastro-intestinal bleeding

Gastro-intestinal haemorrhage will manifest itself through haematemesis; malaena or, more dangerously, through an enlarged abdomen with associated pain. In the latter case, where bleeding occurs into the peritoneum, rather than into the gastro-intestinal tract, the patient may reach the stage of hypovolaemic shock before presenting at the Emergency Department.

The patient presenting with haematemesis may have an underlying gastric or duodenal ulcer or he may have oesophageal varices. Conversely, haematemesis may be the result of injury to the oesophagus or the ingestion (accidental or otherwise) of poisons. Whatever the history, this will be a frightening experience for the patient and is likely to require early surgical intervention. The primary goals of immediate management are to

1 immediately assess for hypovolaemia,
2 find the cause of the haemorrhage,
3 support vital functions to prevent hypoxic or hypovolaemic damage.

Assessment
- Non-invasive assessment of vital signs
- ECG monitoring and 12-lead ECG
- BP – be alert for hypovolaemic shock
- Observe for anxiety – an early sign of shock
- Oxygen saturation
- Blood for U&Es; FBC; clotting screen
- History from relatives: onset, duration and trigger of current symptoms, past history

Immediate interventions
- Fluids as indicated by vital signs
- Oxygen therapy if shocked
- Alert surgeons
- Be alert for cardiac arrest if hypovolaemia is severe
- Prepare the patient and family for the possibility of surgery
- Early endoscopy may be indicated if the cause of the bleeding is unclear.

Fluid replacement

Depending on the extent of the hypovolaemia, the patient may be given a fluid challenge, in order to support the circulation and prevent organ failure. This is often achieved through small repeated boluses of crystalloid or colloid fluid (for example, 200 ml over 10 min). If more than two 200 ml boluses need to be given, the patient must have a CVP line in situ to monitor the effects.

The clinical benefits of colloids over crystalloids are still unclear (Scott 2000). Whilst crystalloid fluid is cheap and provides immediate volume it is rapidly lost from the circulation (up to 75% within 1 hour) through the capillary bed. Colloid fluid such as Gelatins help restore oncotic pressure within the circulation and help prevent capillary leak, but there is an increased risk of anaphylaxis to proteins contained within the fluid. The principle of fluid resuscitation is to increase circulatory volume and provide oxygen-carrying capability. Neither crystalloid nor colloid fluid can carry oxygen therefore in types 3 or 4 early transfusion of blood is highly desirable.

Be aware that CVP may initially remain raised in hypovolaemia due to peripheral vasoconstriction.

If the gastric bleed is due to leaking oesophageal varices, the haemorrhage would be managed more specifically using a Sengstaken tube to put pressure on the bleeding points. The Sengstaken tube is inserted orally into the stomach and balloons inflated to compress the bleeding varices. In addition, traction may be applied to the tube to wedge the inflated balloons against the bottom of the oesophagus. Oesophageal varices are varicosed oesophageal veins that develop as a complication of increased pressure in the portal circulation (portal hypertension). Hence if the varices leak, the blood loss can be severe and fatal. Portal hypertension commonly results from liver disease, hence the patient is likely to have abnormal clotting physiology, adding to the difficulties of managing the haemorrhage.

Gynaecological emergencies

The main gynaecological emergencies which prompt women to present at the Emergency Department are

- abdominal pain,
- vaginal bleeding,
- infections.

The first stage of assessment is to ascertain whether the woman is pregnant, as this will influence both the interpretation of assessment data (for example, heart rate, FBC) and decisions about patient management.

Assessment

- Vital signs – airway, breathing, circulation level of consciousness
- Nature of pain
- Menstrual cycle – date and duration of last menstrual period
- Abnormal vaginal discharge or bleeding
- Medication, including oral contraception
- Past obstetric history
- Urine pregnancy test
- History from relatives: onset, duration and trigger of current symptoms, past history

---

One-sided abdominal pain may indicate the presence of an ovarian cyst. This is a collection of fluid around the corpus luteum, hence pain tends to be worse during the second half of the menstrual cycle. Rupture of a large ovarian cyst may cause severe

hypovolaemic shock, requiring fluid resuscitation and surgical intervention. If the pain can be controlled and the patient has normal vital signs, discharge home is likely, with primary care follow-up and outpatients referral if necessary.

Generalized pelvic pain, not linked to the menstrual cycle, and with accompanying pyrexia, may indicate pelvic inflammatory disease (PID) (infection of the fallopian tubes and ovaries). This is most commonly caused by a sexually transmitted disease and can cause severe problems if the infected area develops an abscess, which may subsequently rupture into the peritoneum. Uncomplicated PID may be managed with antibiotics, with referral to the STD clinic as an outpatient. However, the dangers of abscess formation often necessitate admission for observation and IV antibiotic therapy.

Assessment of the pregnant woman

- BP and pulse – alert for hypovolaemic shock
- Temperature – pyrexia may indicate infection or pre-eclampsia
- Urine analysis for glucose and protein
- Fundal height
- Foetal heart rate (after 16 weeks)
- Type and amount of vaginal loss
- Ultrasound scan
- History of current and previous pregnancies

It should be suspected that the pregnant woman presenting at the Emergency Department with vaginal bleeding is at risk of spontaneous abortion, or miscarriage. Patient-held records assist in identifying the stage and history of current and previous pregnancies, and can enable questioning of the patient to be focused on the presenting problems. Analgesia should be given and IV fluid as indicated by signs of hypovolaemia. If miscarriage seems inevitable, as indicated by amount of blood loss and absence of foetal heartbeat (if foetal gestation is >16 weeks), an ultrasound scan should be undertaken as soon as possible. The woman may have to be prepared for surgery to evacuate retained products if the miscarriage is incomplete.

In a small number of women, in early pregnancy, the fertilized egg will become embedded outside of the endometrium, usually in the fallopian tube. This is known as an *ectopic pregnancy* and may be

Table 4.13
Common forms of metabolic crisis

Crisis	Symptoms	Interventions
Hypoadrenal crisis *Low gluco-corticoid and mineralocorticoid levels* Can be the result of sudden cessation of steroid therapy or periods of extreme stress for patients taking steroids	↓ *Glucocorticoid levels*: Weakness and malaise Vomiting and diarrhoea Abdominal pain Fasting hypoglycaemia ↓ *Mineralocorticoid levels*: Dehydration Sodium deficiency Weight loss Postural hypotension Tachycardia Hyperkalaemia Skin pigmentation (in ACTH excess)	Blood for plasma cortisol levels Manage circulatory failure (hypovolaemia/hypotension) (0.9% saline 1 l over 1 h initially) consider CVP monitoring Resuscitation measures may be necessary Gluco-corticoids to be replenished using hydrocortisone Replacement of deficient mineralocorticoid will only begin after correction of circulatory failure
Thyrotoxic crisis	Diarrhoea vomiting Pyrexia Breathlessness Tachycardia ± tachyarrhythmia Anxiety/psychosis Weight loss Abdominal pain Enlarged thyroid Eyelid retraction	Block thyroid hormone synthesis Block release of thyroid hormone Block effects of circulating thyroid hormones Identify cause (for example, an increase in thyroid-binding proteins – pregnancy; oestrogen treatment; phenothiazine treatment; viral hepatitis)
Myxoedema coma	Depressed level of consciousness Bradycardia Hypotension Hypoventilation Oedema Slow or absent reflexes Hypothermia Hyponatraemia Anaemia Lactic acidosis Seizures	ECG monitoring BM stix Thyroid hormone replacement Resuscitative measures as necessary Correct bradyarrhythmias Transfer to ICU for ventilation, to correct acid–base imbalance and preserve vital functions U&Es – hypoadrenalism is common. Steroids may be necessary

diagnosed at different stages, presenting differing clinical pictures:

1 abdominal pain and intermittent vaginal bleeding;
2 large vaginal bleed, indicating that the embryo has died;
3 sudden abdominal pain and signs of severe hypovolaemic shock, resulting from rupture of the fallopian tube.

At any of these stages, the woman may not have known she was pregnant, particularly if her menstrual cycle is not regular. Hence she may be simultaneously faced with the news that she is (or was) pregnant but that the pregnancy is not viable. Although the possibility of ruptured fallopian tubes makes the condition potentially life threatening, the woman and her partner need to be given time and privacy to come to terms with the diagnosis, if possible. However, intervention for the woman presenting at stage 3 must be prompt as bleeding into the peritoneal cavity cannot be contained without surgery.

Pre-eclampsia

The pregnant woman presenting with hypertension and oedema should be immediately suspected of having pre-eclampsia, or pregnancy induced hypertension. This is a serious, life-threatening condition in which raised BP results in renal impairment, causing proteinuria, and disruption in tissue fluid movement, causing oedema of the face or upper limbs. If the hypertension is not controlled, it will affect other body symptoms, most notably the neurological system, causing visual impairment, headache, seizures and cerebral haemorrhage. The latter two are late signs and indicate eclampsia, which is life threatening to mother and foetus. Seizures should be brought rapidly under control in an attempt to reduce intracerebral pressure and risk of cerebral haemorrhage. Artificial ventilation may be necessary to allow control of seizures and manage pulmonary oedema. Other body systems will rapidly be affected by the hypertension, with acute renal failure, liver damage and disseminated intravascular coagulation (DIC) adding further to the electrolyte and clotting imbalance. The foetus will be delivered urgently, to enable maternal symptoms to be managed more aggressively. Hypertension often reduces following delivery of the foetus. However, other body systems may have become irreparably damaged by the time of delivery and maternal death may follow.

The possible impact of gynaecological problems on a woman's future fertility emphasises the need for sensitive assessment, adequate time for discussion with clinicians and family before surgical intervention and the provision of information to enable fully informed consent for procedures. The need for privacy is emphasised.

THE PATIENT PRESENTING WITH A METABOLIC CRISIS

In addition to disorders of glucose metabolism as discussed earlier, it is important to be aware of the key features and interventions for other metabolic disturbances (see Table 4.13):

References

Adam SK, Osbone S (1997) *Critical care nursing: science and practice*. Oxford: Oxford University Press.

Baskett P, Nolan J (2000) Hypovolaemic shock. In: Driscoll P et al, eds. *ABC of major trauma*, 3rd ed. London: BMJ Publishing Group.

Castledine G (1994) Ethics and the law in A&E. *Emergen Nurs* 2(1): 35.

Davidson J, Hosie H (1993) Limitations of pulse oximetry: respiratory insufficiency – a failure of detection. *Br Med J* 307: 372–373.

Endacott R, Jenks C (1997) Respiratory assessment in A&E. *Emergen Nurs* 5(4): 31–38.

Greaves I, Hodgetts ST, Porter K (1997) *Emergency care: a textbook for paramedics*. London: WB Saunders.

Holt L (2000) Adolescence. In: Dolan B, Holt L, eds. *Accident and emergency: theory into practice*. London: Balliere Tindall.

Kaye P, O'Sullivan I (2002) The role of magnesium in the emergency department. *Emergen Med J* 19(4): 288–291.

Kilner T, Wilkinson R (2000) Medical emergencies. In: Dolan B, Holt L, eds. *Accident and emergency: theory into practice*. London: Balliere Tindall.

King T, Simon R (1987) Pulse oximetry for tapering supplemental oxygen in hospitalised patients. *Chest* 92: 713–716.

Oh TE (1996) *Intensive care manual*, 4th ed. Sydney: Butterworths.

Rooney SJ, Hyde J, Graham T (2000) Chest injuries. In: Driscoll P et al, eds. *ABC of major trauma*, 3rd ed. London: BMJ Publishing Group.

Scott RA (2000) Shock. In: Cameron P, Jelink G, Kelly AM, Murrag L, Heyworth J, eds. *Textbook of adult emergency medicine*. Edinburgh: Churchill Livingstone.

Singer M, Webb AR (1994) *Acute medicine algorithms*. Oxford: Oxford Medical Publications.

Stoneham M (1995) Use and limitations of pulse oximetry. *Br J Hosp Med* 54(1): 35–41.

Thelan LA et al (1990) *Textbook of critical care nursing: diagnosis and management*. St Louis: CV Mosby.

Walthall J (2000) Cardiac emergencies. In: Dolan B, Holt L, eds. *Accident and emergency: theory into practice*. London: Balliere Tindall.

Williams H, Dratcu L, Taylor R, Roberts M, Oyefeso A (1998) "Saturday night fever": ecstasy related problems in a London accident and emergency department. *J Accid Emergen Med* 15(5): 322–326.

Woodrow P (1999) Pulse oximetry. *Nurs Stand* 13(42): 42–46.

5 | Emergency care of the older person

Robert Crouch

This chapter addresses issues around the emergency care of the older person. Common acute conditions or issues that elderly patients present to Emergency Departments with will be explored.

As with other chapters the approach will be structured around body systems and patient symptoms with specific nursing considerations. In addition, issues such as "elder abuse" and the effects of social isolation will be explored.

BACKGROUND

A considerable proportion of the work of the Emergency Department is around older people. In the UK, the proportion of elderly patients (>65 years) who attend the department ranges from 14% to 20% (Bridges et al 1999) and older people now comprise two-thirds of all patients in acute settings (SNMAC 2001a). It is suggested that between 1995 and 2025 the number of people aged over 80 is set to increase by almost a half and that the number over 90 years old will double (DoH 2001). A recent review of the literature around older people in Emergency Department identifies that older people (when compared to younger people) who attend the Emergency Department are more likely to arrive by ambulance; to live alone; to be more acutely ill; to have medical (as opposed to surgical problems) to have significant co-morbidity; spend longer in the department and have more diagnostic tests, and are more likely to be admitted (Bridges et al 1999).

A recent report by the UK Standing Nursing and Midwifery Advisory Committee (SNMAC 2001b) suggests that there are significant deficits in the care provided for older people in the acute setting. These range from failures in the provision of fundamental care

to a lack of specialist educational preparation for nurses caring for older people. The report contains a number of recommendations specifically relating to Emergency Department; these can be found in Figure 5.1.

The recently published National Service Framework for Older People (DoH 2001) sets out ambitious targets for the improvement of care with this group of patients. In particular, targets have been set for improvements in person centred care; intermediate care; general hospital care; stroke; falls; mental health; use of medicines and promoting health, and independence. The NSF and the work of SNMAC focus on the specific needs of the older person. This has been recognized in emergency nursing and specific patient grouping of the older person has been identified as an area where specific competencies and educational preparation are required (Endacott et al 1999). As can been seen from the current and expected demographic picture and the diverse requirements of this patient group, particular attention is warranted for their needs in the emergency setting.

The Royal College of Nursing Emergency Department Association have published a position statement on the older person in Emergency Department (Sowney 1999). In it Sowney states

"Emergency Departments should provide an environment which is appropriate to meet the needs of older people by creating a culture and supporting practice that is respectful of their complex needs, rights, desires, dignity and life experience." (Sowney 1999)

To facilitate a greater understanding of the need to consider more than the presenting complaint, knowledge of the effects of the aging process is required. The following section will outline issues to be considered.

Standard statement: The older person and their carers receive nursing services based on their needs. The assessment process is undertaken by an appropriately qualified person and ensures that services are co-ordinated and delivered across the settings and specialties with which the person may come into contact.

Indicators: People aged 75 years and over are given priority, in terms of their initial assessment and at the point of contact in an Emergency Department situation, e.g. Emergency Department or Medical Admissions Assessment Unit. Target times for their assessment are set and monitored. This assessment should include:

a) baseline information such as the need for interpreting facilities or audio-visual aids;
b) the normal home circumstances of the older person and social support;
c) normal health status;
d) immediate clinical needs.

Specialist nursing advice on care for older people is available to Emergency Department as a minimum standard.

(from *Practice guidance: principles standards and indicators. Caring for older people: a nursing priority.* SNMAC 2001b)

Figure 5.1 Specific statements relating to care of the elderly in Emergency Department

THE AGING PROCESS

As an individual ages there are physiological, sociological and psychological changes. Some of these will be considered in the following sections.

PHYSIOLOGICAL

There are a number of key physiological changes that affect elderly people. These physiological changes often have significant implications for the elderly and should be considered when assessing patients attending the Emergency Department.

Skeletal

■ *Bones*, the shape of long bones alter, becoming thicker due to an increase in the internal cavity but a decrease in thickness of cortical layer leading to a weaker structure.

■ *Loss of bone matrix (reabsorption)* more rapid than bone growth leading to loss of density called osteoporosis. Osteoporosis is more common in women than men.

■ *Reduction in overall physical height* due to shortening of vertebral column (through thinning of intervertebral discs and decrease in height of vertebrae through osteoporosis).

■ *Anterior curvature of the spine (kyphosis)* may develop due to reduced bone size and unequal wasting of musculature around the spine.

■ *Decreased stress tolerance.*

■ *Increased risk of osteomalacia* due to lack of vitamin D leading to recurrent fractures, difficulty walking (including climbing stairs) and constant low back pain. Incidence is thought to be 20–30% of women and 40% of men. Causes are thought to be lack of exposure to sunlight (ultraviolet light is needed to produce vitamin D) and reduced vitamin D uptake from the gut.

■ *Paget's disease* leading to bowing of femora and tibiae caused by an imbalance of bone reabsorption and replacement. Bone turnover can be increased by 20% leading to distortion and weakening of the bone and to secondary problems with associated joints (Barker 1998; Bennett and Ebrahim 1995; Coni and Webster 1998; Jarvis 2000).

■ *Joints*, changes in the structure of synovial fluid affecting joint lubrication and nourishment of articulatory cartilage leading to osteoarthritis – a progressive localized disorder involving the articular cartilages and subchondral bone. Osteophytes, forming new bone at the joint surface may occur. The condition leads to increasing pain and decreased movement. Increase common with increased age but is not a natural consequence of aging and is often related to a secondary cause (Barker 1998; Coni and Webster 1998; Jarvis 2000).

■ *Muscles*, muscle fibre decreases and is replaced by an increase in fat and fibrous tissue leading to a overall reduction in muscle bulk and effectiveness. A 5–7% decrease decline per year for those over 70 years for some muscle groups.

Activity plays an important part in preserving muscle structure. A decrease in muscle mass and tone can affect stability of joints and overall movement and dexterity (Barker 1998; Bennett and Ebrahim 1995; Coni and Webster 1998).

Cardiovascular

There are physiological changes to the cardiovascular system associated with age. Structural changes to the cardiovascular system include: decreased aortic elasticity and widening of the aorta (often seen on X-rays as a widened aortic arch; less mobile heart valves with calcification and age changes to the myocardium with a build-up of a waste product lipofuscin (Bennett and Ebrahim 1995). Pathological changes such as degenerative disease of the heart and associated vessels are common among the elderly and may result in such diseases as

- ischaemic heart disease,
- hypertension,
- valvular disease,
- pulmonary disease,
- cardiomyopathy,
- thyrotoxic effects,
- conducting-tissue disease (Coni and Webster 1998).

Central nervous system and cognitive functioning

It is often difficult to separate out the effects of aging alone on central nervous system from those of disease in the elderly. We do know however that there is a decrease in brain volume and weight associated with aging. There is thought to be a reduction in the number of nerve cells within the brain with older people but no one has ever counted them! We do know that there is no further neurone production after childhood (Ostro 1993). The disappearance of neurones results in a deterioration of response and reaction to sudden stimuli. Impairment in neurotransmission may lead to changes in mood and co-ordination. Memory may also be affected with age, in particular short-term memory. Though it is suggested that the difficulty some older people experience in remembering strings of numbers or lists may

not be associated with age alone rather a consequence of their generation. For instance those who were born in the 1900s had less schooling, less exposure to modern media and less need to remember long strings of numbers for telephones (Bennett and Ebrahim 1995).

SOCIOLOGICAL

There have been many changes in society over the past 50 years, in particular changes in family structure. This change in family structure, from extended to nuclear families, may have resulted in a greater degree of social isolation for a number of older adults. There are cultural differences that need to be considered when assessing the elderly; some cultures place greater emphasis on the importance of older members of the family playing the role of the elder statesperson. Emergency nurses need to develop a cultural awareness of their local population and their views of aging. Illness or injury can also induce social isolation which in turn can have a profound effect on the older person's psychological well-being.

PSYCHOLOGICAL

The physiological effects of aging as detailed in this section may have psychological effects. The older person, may feel little different inside to 20–30 years ago, but may feel constrained and frustrated by physical effects of aging. The loss of a lifetime partner may have profound psychological consequences for the older person leaving them with a loss of will to continue or lack of sense of purpose. Depression is common in the elderly and may manifest in many ways. The psychological consequences of aging should not be underestimated.

ASSESSING THE OLDER PERSON IN THE EMERGENCY DEPARTMENT

As with all aspects of emergency nursing the key to effective care of the older person is assessment.

The assessment must be comprehensive and take account of social, psychological as well as physical factors. The identification of factors leading to their presentation, beyond the seemingly obvious reason, requires a systematic approach. Extra time may be required to discuss concerns. An exploratory study of the experience of older people in Emergency Department identified a lack of opportunity to fully explain their situation to staff (Spilsbury et al 1999). As has already been described, patients may present with multiple pathology. The identification of major concerns such as cancellation of support services or feeding and caring for animals need to be considered. The use of validated assessment tools to explore cognitive and physical function may be a useful adjunct to assessment of the older person. A brief outline will be given in the following section.

ASSESSMENT TOOLS

A tried and tested method of assessment of functional ability is the Barthel Index. The tool is based on observed function and completed by a therapist or observer. It does not measure ability to function in the community, as activities of daily living such as cooking and shopping, and other essential everyday tasks, which limits its application outside the hospital setting (Bowling 1997). All the components listed in the index can be scored in the Emergency Department. Completion of the index will give an indication of functional ability and may help in the decision about safe discharge or the need for further assessment by occupational therapy or referral for admission. The aspects of daily living covered by the scale are shown in Figure 5.2.

The scale for the assessment of cognitive ability is the Abbreviated Mental Test Score (AMTS). This tool is not designed to diagnose dementia, but rather to assess the cognitive ability of the older person. This assessment is useful in taking decisions about safe discharge

or the need for referral for further assessment. The scale has ten items; a correct answer attracts a score of 1, giving a maximum score of 10. The range of scores which determines normal cognitive ability vary in the literature (Bowling 1997), however a useful guide is provided by Bowman (1997): 0–3, severe impairment; 4–7, moderate impairment; 8–10, normal. The 10 items contained in the test are shown in Figure 5.3.

There are many other validated tests that may be useful. A guide to validated tests can be found in Bowling (1997).

An essential component of assessment is communication. Effective communication with the older adult is fundamental; consideration should be given to specific challenges presented by the aging process, in particular the possibility of impaired hearing and eyesight. This may necessitate providing access to aids for communication as well as addressing signage in the department. Basic steps should be taken to ensure that hearing aids that are in place are functioning and that you ascertain the best side to approach or communicate with the patient.

Communication also includes significant others. In the care of the older person, with their consent, relatives or significant others should be included in the assessment of the older person, planning of care and transfer or discharge from the department.

It is essential to remember that the older person has less physiological reserve because of aging, drug therapy and co-morbidity (Ritchie 2000). This may result in an altered or unpredictable presentation to a younger adult suffering the same injury or illness.

Perhaps the assessment of older person in Emergency Department can be captured by the maxim – *If you aren't looking for it you won't find it!*

Feeding
Mobility from bed to chair
Getting off the toilet
Grooming
Bathing
Walking on level surfaces
Going up- and downstairs
Dressing
Continence (bladder and bowel)

Figure 5.2 Aspects of daily living included in the Barthel Index

Age
Time (to nearest hour)
Year
Name of place
Recognition of two persons
Birthday (date and month)
Date of World War 1
Name of present monarch
Counting 20–1 backwards
Five-minute recall: full address of patient should be asked and then asked again in 5 min

Figure 5.3 The ten items of the Abbreviated Mental Test

Robert Crouch

AGE-SPECIFIC CONSIDERATIONS WITH CLINICAL PRESENTATIONS

The following section will address some of the age-specific clinical presentations to the Emergency Department.

CEREBRAL VASCULAR ACCIDENT

One of the common presentations associated with the older person, although not exclusive to, is that of a cerebral vascular accident (CVA). It is defined as "focal neurological deficit of vascular origin which lasts >24 h" (Wyatt et al 1999). Each year 110,000 people have their fist stroke, 30,000 people go on to have further strokes (DoH 2001). There are two principle mechanisms of CVA, infarction or haemorrhage with the incidence being 80% and 20%, respectively. As new approaches to early treatment are being trialed with the aim of reversing occlusion and therefore reducing the damage of infarction the exploration of the mechanism is becoming increasingly important (Wyatt et al 1999).

The Emergency Department has a role to play in both the initial treatment of patient's presenting with a CVA and in the possible prevention of CVA. The preventative role is one of general health education in particular the role of hypertension in stroke.

As a routine for many presentations in the Emergency Department the patient's blood pressure will be recorded. An elevated reading should not be ignored. Consideration should be given to likely causes, such as stress or pain as well as other physiological causes relating to their presenting complaint. The discovery of an elevated blood pressure may be co-incidental and although a single elevated reading does not confirm hypertension it should either be repeated in the Emergency Department or the patient advised to visit their GP for follow-up. The asymptomatic nature of hypertension means that it has been labelled a silent killer (Getliffe et al 2000); the visit to the Emergency Department may be the only time that the patient's blood pressure has been checked for a number of years. Other health education about diet and exercise can also be given.

Immediate care of the patient presenting with a CVA is presented below for the general approach see Figure 5.4.

Immediate care of the patient with a CVA

Assessment

- *Airway*
  - Patency of the airway
  - Any dysphagia?
- *Breathing*
  - Rate and depth – consider adequacy
  - Record SaO_2
  - Chest auscultation
- *Circulation*
  - By definition of the CVA there has been an insult on the circulation
  - Heart rate, blood pressure, ECG, BM
- *Disability*
  - Record full Glasgow Coma Score (GCS)
- *Exposure*
  - Any injuries, signs of trauma
  - Record core temperature

Interventions

- Consider airway positioning and the use of adjuncts such as oro-pharangeal/ naso-pharangeal airway if airway compromised
- Suctioning should be available
- High flow oxygen to aid cerebral perfusion
- Intravenous access should be secured
- Nurse patient on the side, take care when positioning affected limbs not to compromise circulation
- ECG to check underlying rhythm, specifically looking for atrial fibrillation
- Psychological support for both patient and relatives/significant others
- Continuous observation – risk of extending stroke and deterioration
- Record blood sugar

FALL

Attendance at the Emergency Department following a fall is common. Although the death rate associated with falls is on the decline overall, this is not the case for older people (DoH 1998). There are significant costs associated with falling in physical, psychological and economic terms to the individual, their family and society as a whole. There have been many epidemiological studies exploring risk factors for

Emergency care of the older person

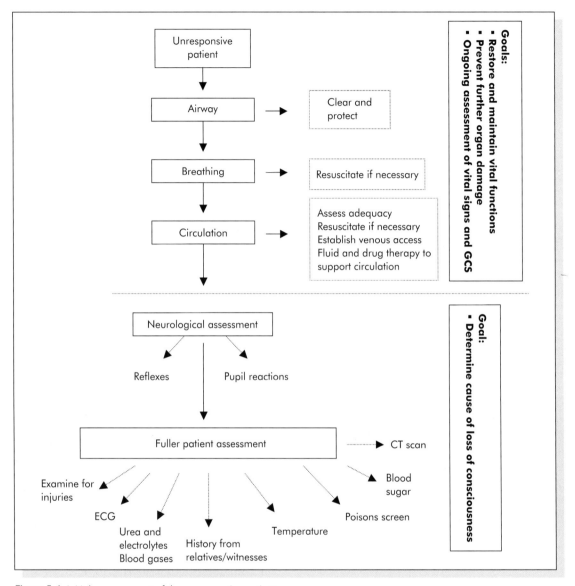

Figure 5.4 Initial management of the unresponsive patient

falling. The most frequently cited risk factors are shown in Table 5.1 (Effective Health Care 1996)

Four factors have been found to be predictive of recurrent falls in older people (Tromp et al 2001):

> **Four key factors in predicting recurrent falls**
> - Previous falls
> - Urinary incontinence
> - Visual impairment
> - Benzodiazepine use

A systematic and in-depth assessment of the older patient who has fallen is required in the Emergency Department. A crucial first stage in this assessment is confirmation that this was a fall, and not the result of a subtle collapse. The following maxim may be useful in remembering this:

> *"A fall is only a fall after a collapse has been ruled out."*

Robert Crouch

Table 5.1
Potential risk factors

Nutritional status	Environmental hazards	Medication	Lack of exercise	Age-related changes/medical conditions
Deficiency of vitamin D and calcium	Including loose carpets, poor lighting, baths without handles, unsafe stairways	In particular psychotropic agents, polypharmacy, certain cardiovascular drugs (particularly vasodilators) (Hanlon et al 1996)	Associated with muscle weakness, poor gait and balance and accelerated bone loss	Deterioration of vision, cognitive impairment

Older patients attending the Emergency Department with any of the risk factors identified in above and in Table 5.1 should trigger extra concern and action considered providing more in-depth assessment of risk to prevent further falls. Referral for assessment by an occupational therapist, whose prime role is to promote independent function, should be considered. The effect of the fall on the individual's self-confidence should not be underestimated. Referral to other agencies and the provision of support/equipment in the home may only go a small way to restoring this. Self-confidence should be considered when assessing suitability for discharge. Another important component of assessment is eliciting corroborative information about the person and their ability to cope. Fabrication of the ability to cope is not uncommon; information should be sought (with permission from the patient) from relatives, GP and other social networks as appropriate. Sensitivity is fundamental in the assessment of the older person as they may have insight into their needs but there can be an understandable reluctance to admit that they are having difficulty coping or feel vulnerable.

The assessment of the older patient who has fallen is complex; the following acronym based on the word FALLS (see Figure 5.5, p. 82) provides a framework for use in the Emergency Department.

As can be seen from Figure 5.5, the assessment of the older person who has fallen should be systematic and comprehensive. This often presents a challenge in a busy Emergency Department. Elements of the assessment could be conducted by the emergency nurse whilst many areas can be referred to other professional groups specializing in the assessment of activities of daily living, rehabilitation and social support.

The older person who has fallen may feel vulnerable, embarrassed that they are a burden or humiliated. Their reaction to your questioning may appear inappropriate or ungrateful. The effect of the fall on their loss of self-esteem and confidence should not be underestimated, and considerable tact and diplomacy in questioning and assessment are fundamental.

FRACTURED NECK OF FEMUR

This injury is not isolated to the older person but it is certainly more common amongst this group. Hip fractures are three times more likely in women than in men (Wyatt et al 1999). This injury is usually caused by a fall or collapse, and is likely to cause significant distress to the individual as well as physical pain. Although a common presentation, there is significant scope for improvement of care. Although generally considered to be a non-life threatening injury, there may be significant co-morbidity; complications of the injury and resultant incapacitation should be considered.

The characteristics of the typical presentation are shown below.

The typical presentation of a fractured neck of femur

- History of fall or collapse with impact on the lateral aspect of the hip
- Pain in the groin with/without radiation to the knee
- Pain exacerbated by movement
- Usually unable to weight bear (although do not be fooled, with an impacted fracture the patient may be able to mobilize with difficulty!)

Emergency care of the older person

F – Falls history
Time (including time on the ground); location; mechanism (including exploration of hazards); loss of conscious/ lack of recollection; method of raising alarm/rescue and frequency/pattern of falls.

A – Assessment
As previously stated it is essential to rule out collapse as a cause of the fall. The fundamentals of emergency care should be observed namely: Airway; Breathing; Circulation; Disability (full neurological assessment) and Exposure (a full physical assessment is required to determine extent of injuries and co-morbidity). Core body temperature (hypothermia may be a consequence/cause of a fall). Postural hypotension should be explored. Injury/ illness – need to explore and document possible causes and effects of the fall. Risk factors/assessment for fall and or re-current falls and suitability of return to home. Referral for full assessment by occupational therapist/social services. Environmental causes should be explored such as trip hazards should be assessed. Nutritional status and drug history. Explore effects of change in capability of the older person on others, i.e. dependents/carers.

L – Locomotor problems
The physiological effects of aging should be considered. Assessment of the joint movement and stability of both lower and upper limbs should be undertaken. Observation of walking and movement from a sitting to walking position should be undertaken. Posture, stance and gait should also be considered.

L – Loss
Loss of or reduced vision is a known risk factor for falls. Visual acuity should be assessed and recorded. Assessment should include the consideration of cataracts, macular degeneration, glaucoma, diabetic retinopathy. Poor lighting is a consideration and should be explored in conjunction with visual loss as a contributing environmental factor. Loss of self-confidence is common after a fall. This must be acknowledged and efforts made to offer support and practical advice that can be followed to help prevent falls in the future. This may include referral to social services or voluntary support services.

S – Social circumstances
History of social circumstances – living alone; carer; dependents; recent bereavement. Support network relatives (formal) or friends (informal). Type of housing and suitability. Social contact.

Figure 5.5 FALLS – The assessment of the older person who has fallen

- Displacement at the fracture site may result in the classic shortened and rotated affected limb – beware this may not always be the case

There are a number of potential complications of the injury and the resultant incapacitation:

Potential complications

1 *Avascular necrosis of the head of femur*: the medial and lateral circumflex femoral arteries provide the blood supply to the head and neck of femur. The medial circumflex femoral artery is often disrupted with fracture of the femoral neck which may dramatically reduce blood supply to the head of femur.

2 *Hypovolaemia or dehydration*: resulting in reduced circulatory volume. Although large volume blood loss is not normally associated with neck of femur fractures, this should be considered until definitive diagnosis as large volume loss is associated with intertrochanteric and shaft of femur fractures. Dehydration may be as a result of prolonged isolation/immobilization after a fall.

3 *Skin integrity*: consideration should be given to skin integrity of pressure areas. The patient will naturally want to splint their injury which may lead to a reluctance to move. Care should be taken to prevent the breakdown of pressure areas.

The initial management and investigations of a patient with a suspected fractured neck of femur are shown on the next page.

The differential assessment of the older person who has fallen should include dislocation of the hip. The symptoms may mimic a fractured neck of femur. With a typical posterior dislocation (accounting for 90% of non-prosthetic dislocations, Holt 2000), the hip may be held flexed, adducted and internally rotated. The leg may appear shorter. This presentation

---

Initial management and investigation of a patient with a suspected fractured neck of femur

Airway	Open and maintain
Breathing	Consider supplementary oxygen if low SpO$_2$ (beware contraindications of O$_2$ therapy)
	Continuous SpO$_2$ monitoring (caution consider peripheral perfusion)
Circulation	Assess for signs/indications of haemorrhage
	Check circulation distal to fracture
	Capillary refill
	Consider avascular necrosis of head of femur
	Consider intravenous fluid replacement and for the prevention of dehydration if to be nil by mouth
Pain	Intravenous route opiod analgesia (titrated regularly to pain)
	Intravenous anti-emetic
	Check for any alteration in sensation distal to fracture
	Position of the leg may also help to reduce pain, consider the prevention of further external rotation which may increase muscle spasm
	NB: The routine use of skin traction pre-operatively is not advocated (Considine and Hood 2000)
Investigations	X-ray hip and pelvis
	Bloods – urea and electrolytes, full blood count (FBC), group and save, glucose
	12-lead ECG to rule out cardiac abnormalities as a cause of fall and as a routine pre-operatively
Pressure area relief	Consider pressure relieving mattress
	Pressure area relief every 30 min
Referral	Early referral is advocated to orthopaedic team
	Integrated care pathways or fast track pathways should be followed where they exist

---

is associated with extreme pain, pain may be less severe however if the acetabulum is fractured. The presentation may be concealed if there is a fracture of the shaft of femur. The mechanism of injury includes high impact trauma such as a fall from a height or an RTA (particularly when the knee hits the dashboard. In an anterior dislocation of the hip the leg is usually held in abduction and is shortened and rotated. Swelling and bruising may be seen in the groin (Holt 2000; McRae 1999).

Early reduction of a traumatic dislocation of a hip is essential in reducing pain and preventing complications. Complications associated with traumatic dislocation include – sciatic nerve palsy; avascular necrosis of the femoral head; femoral artery or vein compression and femoral nerve paralysis (in particular with anterior dislocations) (McRae 1999).

Points to remember

It may be a common injury to you, but probably the first time for the patient

Although not immediately life threatening – the long-term threat to mortality from complications is significant

"OFF THEIR LEGS"

This is a common catchall term used to describe a general deterioration of an individual. Although it can have pejorative connotations it requires significant attention in terms of assessment – beneath this benign description may be significant physical and/or psychological pathology. The assessment of

Respiratory	*Assessment* – respiratory rate, peak flow, percussion and auscultation of lung fields, monitor SaO_2, blood gas *Consider* – hypoxia, hypercapnia, hypercapnia encephalopathy, exacerbation of COPD, chest infection or pneumonia, heamoptysis
Cardiovascular	*Assessment* – pulse rate and character, ECG, central and peripheral pulses, capillary refill, blood pressure *Consider* – cardiac arrhythmia (particularly atrial fibrillation and associated risk of microemboli), cardiomyopathy, atherosclerosis particularly of carotid arteries
Digestive	*Assessment* – hydration (skin turgor, state of tongue and other mucous membranes), nutritional state (general appearance, fit of clothes, history and signs of recent weight loss), ability to swallow, vomiting, colour of skin and sclera, bowel habit, alcohol consumption *Consider* – dehydration, malnutrition, change in bowel habit (diarrhoea, constipation, melaena), dysphagia, haematemesis, biliary tract disease
Neurology	*Assessment* – level of consciousness (GCS, full neurological assessment: pupils, limb strengths, blood pressure, pulse), orientation – (Abbreviated Mental Test), history of, or signs of, trauma, dysphasia or dysphagia *Consider* – TIA, CVA, head injury, intra-cranial bleed, meningitis, dementia, new onset confusion, post-ictal
Genitourinary	*Assessment* – urine output, urine sample (for macro and microscopic examination), body temperature recording *Consider* – urinary tract infection, acute renal failure, urinary retention
Endocrine	*Assessment* – blood sugar, pulse rate, temperature, urinalysis *Consider* – diabetes mellitus, thyroid and adrenal emergencies, diabetic ketoacidosis
Metabolic	*Assessment* – state of hydration (skin turgor, state of tongue and other mucous membranes), blood samples for electrolytes and blood gas analysis *Consider* – dehydration, electrolyte disturbance, acid–base disorder such as metabolic acidosis/alkalosis
Haematology	*Assessment* – as for cadiovascular, including close examination of skin for signs of purpura or rash, body temperature, history of, or signs of, trauma *Consider* – anaemia, haemorrhage, neutropenia
Psychiatric	*Assessment* – general physical state (clothing/cleanliness), delirium, hallucinations, altered mood, demeanor, affect, eye contact, orientation and understanding – physical causes of the above should be ruled out. Consider using a validated depression index *Consider* – depression, anxiety, panic attack, overdose, elder abuse, self-neglect
Other	*Assessment* – general state, unaccounted injuries, GCS *Consider* – hypothermia, elder abuse

Figure 5.6 Areas for consideration in the assessment of the older person who is describes as "off their legs"

the older person should be carried out in conjunction with their "significant others".

A systematic approach is recommended for assessment; there is no right or wrong approach a systems approach is adopted in the following areas for consideration (see Figure 5.6).

LOSS OF CONSCIOUSNESS

An elderly patient presenting with loss of consciousness or a reduced GCS is not uncommon. There are many reasons for loss of consciousness; a systematic approach to assessment is essential when seeking to determine the cause. In terms of initial assessment and intervention the principles of Airway, Breathing and Circulation should be applied, for the general approach see Figure 5.4 (p. 80). Endocrine emergencies should be explored such as hypo- or hyperglycaemia; hypothyroidism as should neurological causes for the loss of consciousness such as CVAs; trans-ischaemic attacks (see Chapter 4) and trauma (see Chapter 7).

Airway and breathing	Consider respiratory rate and effectiveness. Percuss and auscultate lung fields for signs of wheeze, consolidation and failure. Consider hypoxia; hypercapnia; CO poisoning, SaO_2 monitoring and blood gas analysis. Consider acute exacerbation of COPD.
Circulation	ECG, consider cardiac causes; arrhythmias; failure; infection. Consider hydration, skin turgor, urea and electrolyte imbalance (particular hyponatraemia due to diuretics for treating cardiac failure), anaemia (FBC). Record pulse, blood pressure.
Disability	Full GCS and neurological observations, consider neurological causes. Hypoglycaemia, BM and laboratory blood sugar. Consider cognitive ability, use an established tool for assessing cognitive ability such as Abbreviate Mental Test.
Exposure	Full examination, consider hidden trauma, evidence of neglect (nutritional status), self-harm or abuse?
History	Involve others in eliciting the history, family, friends, neighbours, ambulance crew, GP, etc. Consider normal activities of daily living.
Past medical history	Consider if this an exacerbation of a chronic problem, or as consequence of withdrawal of treatment.
Medication	Consider if the confusional state is a result of polypharmacy or accidental/deliberate overdose or poor compliance.
Other investigations	Record temperature, consider hypothermia. Pyrexia, screen for infection; urine, sputum, wounds, take and test relevant samples including blood cultures.

Figure 5.7 Assessment of the patient with an acute confusional state

One of the common reasons for presentation with loss of consciousness in elderly is hypothermia (for management of hypothermia see Chapter 4). In the older person it is important to ascertain whether the hypothermia is precipitant or a consequence of other pathology. Hypothermia alone is a major cause of mortality amongst the older population every year.

Cardiovascular causes of a sudden loss of consciousness examples include arrhythmias, in particular atrial fibrillation with the associated risk of microemboli and postural hypotension.

As with any patient with a history of sudden loss of consciousness (collapse) the routine of investigation should include the recording of respiratory rate and effort, pulse, blood pressure, temperature, ECG, full neurological assessment, blood sugar, urea and electrolytes.

CONFUSION

A confusional state should never be assumed to be a natural consequence of the aging process or immediately related to dementia. The incidence of dementia in the elderly (>80 years) increases but only to above 2%, therefore the majority of elderly patients attending the department will not be demented (although dementia may lead to an increase in attendance for the individual) (Bowman 1997). A confusional state is a broad grouping; reasons for the state can include neurological, metabolic (including endocrine and electrolyte imbalance), cardiovascular and respiratory, infection, psychological and psychiatric. As identified earlier in this chapter, there are a number of physiological changes related to aging that make the achievement and sustainability of homeostasis a constant challenge. A simple urinary tract infection may have significant consequences for the older person. The assessment of the older person with a confusional state must include others who have previous knowledge of the person, relatives, friends/neighbours and the GP.

A guide to the assessment of the older patient presenting with an acute confusional state is given in Figure 5.7.

One of the fundamental issues to address with this type of patient in the Emergency Department is that of environmental safety. The acute confusional state renders the individual vulnerable to numerous hazards within the department and they will be highly dependent on nursing staff for observation and care. A multi-agency approach is advocated for the assessment of the older person with an acute confusional state. There are two key approaches to management:

1 elimination or correction of underlying aetiological disturbances,
2 the provision of symptomatic and supportive care (Dolan 2000).

PAIN

Pain is not a natural consequence of aging and should not be "lived with". The fundamental principle of identify the root cause of the pain should be adopted. The principles of pain management should be equally applied to this older person which includes, if necessary, the administration of opiates. As with all age groups administration should be titrated to pain rather than administration of a pre-prescribed bolus.

There are physiological changes related to aging that affect the peripheral nervous system. However, it is not clear whether this leads to a lack of recognition of pain or to underreporting due to the development of coping strategies (Davis 2000). Whether it is a lack of recognition of pain or a advanced coping strategies, a heightened awareness of the possibility of significant undiagnosed pathology, which would usually be evident when associated with significant pain, analgesia is required.

There may be particular challenges faced by the older person with dementia or confusion in expressing pain. In addition the assessment of pain in the older person may require additional or different assessment strategies than for younger adults (Davis 2000).

MALNUTRITION

Malnutrition may be a contributory or precipitating factor to illness or injury resulting in presentation to the Emergency Department. Assessment of nutritional state is important in determining, firstly whether malnutrition is a contributory or causative factor and secondly in recognizing, and making provision for, the increased nutrients and energy required for healing.

Malnutrition can be a contributing factor to hypothermia, decreased muscle bulk, leading to immobility and ataxia making the individual more susceptible to falls and injury (Hughes 1997). The onset of malnutrition may be insidious and may not be immediately apparent to the individual or their relatives or friends. Indeed the individual may still be eating or drinking; but this may just be what is to hand such as tea and biscuits and not a balanced meal. There are numerous reasons for malnutrition for example: lack of money; difficulty getting to the shops; decreased mobility; difficulty swallowing due to a recent medical problem such as a CVA; malabsorption of food due a clinical condition; lack of skill in preparation and cooking of food; lack of understanding about food types and the need for a balanced diet; ill-fitting dentures; loneliness – suddenly having to cook or feed one after the death of a spouse or loved one; depression or loss of appetite as a side effect of medication (Jarvis 2000).

The identification of malnutrition or the potential for malnutrition should be considered in the overall assessment of the older person in Emergency Department. Social services and the community/hospital dietetics services should have a major role to play in ensuring that sufficient provision is made in the community on discharge. The role of the emergency nurse is to identify the actual or potential problem and refer for specialist intervention.

In assessing the nutritional state of the older person the questions/observations in Figure 5.8 may be helpful; as always considerable tact and diplomacy is required to ensure that no offence is caused by asking such questions.

Observations
  Do they look malnourished – overly thin, history of
    weight loss, are clothes ill fitting?
  Muscle bulk, poor muscle tone?
  Loss of skin turgor?
  Loss of hair?

Questions
  Do you get hungry for your meals?
  What do you normally eat in a day?
  When did you last have a hot meal?
  How many hot meals a week do you have?
  Are you able to cook for yourself?
  Are you able to shop for yourself?
  Do they have a clinical or psychological problem
    that is causing difficulties?

Figure 5.8 Questions/observations to be considered in nutritional assessment

Signs and symptoms of dehydration
- Increased thirst
- Loss of skin elasticity (turgor)
- Dry mucous membranes
- Sunken eyes
- Decreased and concentrated urinary output
- (not in the case of excessive diuresis caused by diabetes or induced by diuretics)
- Hypotension
- Tachycardia
- Increased respiratory rate
- Acute weight loss

Assessment
- *History*: full history of events including when last ate and drank reason for attendance, past medical and drug history
- *Airway*: check patency
- *Breathing*: assess rate and depth of respiration, percussion and auscultation (for signs of pulmonary oedema), pulse oximetry and blood gas analysis dependent upon respiratory findings
- *Circulation*: pulse rate and characteristics, check blood pressure, check blood sugar, cannulation and venesection (urea and electrolytes, FBC, clotting)
- *Disability*: level of consciousness
- *Exposure*: examine body particularly skin turgor, mucous membranes, eyes; check body temperature
- *Other*: check urinary output, take sample and for testing

Figure 5.9 Guide to the identification of dehydration and the assessment of the patient with suspected dehydration

DEHYDRATION

As with malnutrition there are many causes and consequences of dehydration in the older person. It is likely that the state of dehydration will be identified through assessment.

When assessing hydration and exploring possible causes, non-pathological or physiological causes should be explored. The possibility of self-induced, accidental dehydration with the older person should be considered. Increased frequency of micturition in the elderly, particularly at night, combined with increased difficulty with mobilization may lead the individual to severely limit their fluid intake to reduce the number of trips to the toilet.

Dehydration may be as complication of prescribed medication such as diuretics, which (with specific diuretics) may in turn lead to significant electrolyte imbalance such as hyponatraemia or hypokalaemia. As well as depletion through withholding or difficulty accessing fluids or through increased dieresis (chemical, diabetes mellitus/insipidous, urinary tract infection) other causes include, diarrhoea and vomiting, burns or haemorrhage.

Care should be taken with re-hydration. Given the patho-physiological changes associated with aging, rapid re-hydration may cause excess strain on the heart resulting in a degree of cardiac failure resulting in pulmonary and or peripheral oedema.

A guide to the identification of dehydration and the assessment of the patient with suspected dehydration can be found in Figure 5.9.

POLYPHARMACY

As has been indicated throughout this chapter medication, the volume and or the combination of medications, may be a contributory or causative factors in illness or injury with older people, this can be referred to as iatrogenic injury or illness. Polypharmacy is a term used to denote multiple combinations of drug therapies.

The older patient presenting to the Emergency Department often arrives with a container full of medications, sometimes the medications are separated from their packaging and are presented in boxes detailed for different times of day and days of week! The "pill box" is sometimes received with a degree of loathing but in fact may contain a wealth of information useful for assessment and diagnosis. When assessing the older patient attending the department following an injury or illness the following maxim and sentence may be useful to remember in your assessment:

> *Is it a "pill" that has caused this "ill"?*
>
> Did they trip over their pill (falls induced by medication) or just drop their pressure (postural hypotension – complication of treatment of heart failure and hypertension), is their heart too slow (digoxin toxicity – risk of arrhythmias, effects of beta-blockers), or are they too dry to swallow (over diuresis, electrolyte imbalance) or are they confused by the array of medications (drug-induced confusion)?

Careful examination and documentation of its contents and discussion with the patient, about when which medications are taken and what for (to elicit their understanding) is fundamental. Another key individual in this process is the family doctor/practitioner and pharmacist.

Prescribing and administration of medication to the older person requires particular experience and expertise. Fundamental to safe prescribing and administration is an understanding of the physiological changes associated with aging (see earlier sections of this chapter). A secondary check of the side effects, interactions, cautions and dose recommendations for medications prescribed in the Emergency Department is highly recommended.

If medication is suspected as the cause or a contributing factor to the injury or illness the natural temptation is to stop the offending medication. This decision should not be taken in isolation; the patient's usual doctor should be involved in the decision (Bowman 1997).

ELDER ABUSE

Elder abuse is an emotive subject but one that has to be confronted by emergency nurses. Estimates of the prevalence of elder abuse are problematic given the differences in definitions used and the difficulty in extrapolating evidence from research to the general population (McCreadie 1996). This is compounded by the fact that Emergency Department staff do not routinely screen for elder abuse nor is data on it routinely captured. The true extent of elder abuse may never be discovered, however, it should be considered as a

cause of presentation amongst the elderly. Indeed the same principles apply to elder abuse as they do to child abuse, there should be a high index of suspicion when the history or mechanism does not match the injury or illness presented.

The different forms of abuse applying to adults (>18 years, including the elderly) include:

- *physical*, including hitting, slapping, pushing, kicking, misuse of medication, restraint, or inappropriate sanction;
- *sexual*, including rape and sexual assault or sexual acts to which the vulnerable adult has not consented, or could not consent or was pressured into consenting;
- *psychological*, including emotion abuse, threats to harm or abandonment, deprivation of contact, humiliation, blaming, controlling, intimidation, coercion, harassment, verbal abuse, isolation or withdrawal from services or supportive networks;
- *financial or material*, including theft, fraud, exploitation, pressure in connection with wills, property or inheritance or financial transactions, or the misuse or misappropriation of property, possessions or benefits;
- *neglect and acts omission*, including ignoring medical or physical care needs; failure to provide access appropriate health, social care or educational services, the withholding of the necessities of life, such as medication, adequate nutrition and heating; and
- *discriminatory*, including racist, sexist, that based on a person's disability, and other forms of harassment, slurs or similar treatment (DoH 2000).

INTERVENTION IN ELDER ABUSE

The following acronym, END ABUSE, may be useful as an aide memoire for intervention when elder abuse is suspected (see Figure 5.10).

DEPRESSION IN THE ELDERLY

Although depression should be in the hierarchy of causes for consideration when assessing an older person, it should not be near the top. It is not a natural consequence of the aging process. As has been seen in

Empowerment – enable people to know what their choices are, the choices need to be feasible and practical (information should be made available and known by staff in advance).

Neglect – neglect is a much a form of abuse as a violent act. This may be the only sign when identified it requires action.

Documentation – careful documentation of injury and or illnesses is essential for future reference if legal action is to be taken. Remember to document the patient's own words.

Advocacy – in the case of a vulnerable elderly person who is either physically or mentally incapacitated, and are unable to speak for themselves you may have to act as their advocate.

Be aware – aware of the agencies that can assist and have information that can be given to the victim to hand (this may need to be discreet as they).

Understanding – part of the intervention is to help the victim to understand that abuse is a crime, that they are a victim (it is not their fault) and that help is available.

Social services – early involvement of social services is essential when abuse is identified.

Education – education of staff in the recognition of elder abuse and the sensitive steps to be taken when identified is fundamental.

Figure 5.10 END ABUSE – a guide to intervention

other sections of this chapter it does feature in a number of clinical presentations, but it may not be the principle cause of the presenting features; there is a temptation to label an older person as depressed. For instance there may be other chronic illness such as hypothyroidism or hypokalaemia that may mimic depression. As in other aspects of assessment of the older person, the involvement of other people who know the patient (with consent) is essential in gathering an adequate history.

Physical causes should be explored before the diagnosis of depression is made. When the diagnosis is made a careful risk assessment should be performed to assess safety for discharge or referral for admission or specialist opinion (see Chapter 6, Care Plan 2 for a useful risk assessment framework). Good liaison with the local department of psychiatry, social services and voluntary agencies is essential in ensuring a safety net available in the community for those patients who are discharged.

CURRENT PRESSURES AND FUTURE TRENDS

Care of the older person in the Emergency Department is an area that has received little attention in the past; given the burgeoning elderly population, specialist knowledge and education in this area is of increasing importance. The provision of social and community care is inadequate to meet the current needs of the aging population, particularly in what is notionally called the out-of-hours period. This is an international phenomenon, resulting in many elderly patients being nursed in inappropriate environments. The emergency nurse has a key role in identifying gaps in service provision and where such gaps exist, notifying the agencies concerned. Similarly the emergency nurse has a key role to play in identifying health care needs. The needs identified however, are likely to be multi-factorial including social care needs such as practical help with shopping or cooking; practical needs such as alterations to homes to make the environment safe and mobility needs such as the use of mobility aids. To effectively meet these needs early referral to the specialist multi-disciplinary team is fundamental.

CONCLUSION

This chapter has covered the physiological effects of aging and a number of common reasons for presentation of the older person. In-depth assessment of the eldery person is essential in identifying and treating co-morbidity. In the elderly things rarely happen in isolation, anticipation of the consequences and effects of injury and illness, physiologically, sociologically and psychologically are keys to effective emergency care of the older person.

Emergency care of the older person

References

Barker K (1998) The aging process. In: Marr J, Kershaw B, eds. *Caring for older people – developing specialist practice*. London: Arnold.

Bennett GC, Ebrahim S (1995) *Health care in old age*, 2nd ed. London: Arnold.

Bowling A (1997) *Measuring health – a review of quality of life measurement scales*, 2nd ed. Buckingham: Open University Press.

Bowman C (1997) Care of the elderly. In: Skinner D, Swain A, Peyton R, Robertson C, eds. *Cambridge textbook of accident and emergency medicine*. Cambridge: Cambridge University Press.

Bridges J, Spilsbury K, Meyer J, Crouch R (1999) Older people in A&E: literature review and implications for British policy and practice. *Rev Clin Gerentol* 9: 127–137.

Coni N, Webster S (1998) *Lecture notes on geriatrics*, 5th ed. Oxford: Blackwell Science.

Considine J, Hood K (2000) Emergency department management of hip fractures: development of an evidence-based clinical guideline by literature review and consensus. *Emergen Med* 12: 329–336.

Davis BD (2000) *Caring for people in pain*. London: Routledge.

Department of Health (1998) *Saving lives. Our healthier nation. A contract for health*. Department of Health: HMSO Publications.

Department of Health (2000) *No secrets: guidance on developing and implementing multi-agency policies and procedures to protect vulnerable adults from abuse*. London: Department of Health.
http://www.doh.gov.uk/scg/nosecrets.htm

Department of Health (2001) *National service framework for older people*. London: Department of Health.

Dolan B (2000) The eldery. In: Dolan B, Holt L, eds. *Accident and emergency theory into practice*. Edinburgh: Balliere Tindall.

Effective Health Care (1996) *Preventing falls and subsequent injury in older people*, vol. 2(4): Glasgow: Churchill Livingstone.

Endacott R, Edwards B, Crouch R, Castille K, Dolan B, Hamilton C, Jones G, MacPhee D, Manley K, Windle J (1999) Towards a faculty of emergency nursing. *Emergen Nurs* 7(5): 10–16.

Getliffe K, Crouch R, Gage H, Lake F, Wilson S (2000) Hypertension awareness, detection and treatment in a University community: results of a work-site screening. *Public Health* 114: 361–366.

Hughes G (1997) Trauma in the elderly. In: Skinner D, Swain A, Peyton R, Robertson C, eds. *Cambridge textbook of accident and emergency medicine*. Cambridge: Cambridge University Press.

Holt L (2000) Skeletal injuries. In: Dolan B, Holt L, eds. *Accident and emergency theory into practice*. Edinburgh: Balliere Tindall.

Jarvis C (2000) *Physical examination and health assessment*, 3rd ed. Philadelphia: W.B. Saunders.

McRae R (1999) *Pocket book of orthopaedics and fractures*. London: Churchill Livingstone.

McRaedie C (1996) *Elder abuse: update on research*. London: Age Concern Institute of Gerontology, King's College London.

Ostro M (1993) Care of the elderly person. In: Hincliff SM, Norman SE, Schober JE, eds. *Nursing practice and healthcare*, 2nd ed. London: Edward Arnold.

Ritchie P (2000) Trauma in the elderly. In: Cameron P, Jelineck G, Kelly A, Murray L, Heyworth J, eds. *Textbook of adult emergency medicine*. Sydney: Churchill Livingstone.

Sowney R (1999) Older people in A&E – a position statement. *Emergen Nurs* 7(6): 6–7.

Splisbury K, Meyer J, Bridges J, Holman C (1999) Older adults experience of A&E care. *Emergen Nurs* 7(6): 24–31.

SNMAC, Standing Nursing and Midwifery Advisory Committee (2001a) Caring for older people: a nursing priority. Integrating knowledge, practice and values. *Report of the Nursing and Midwifery Advisory Committee*. London: Department of Health.

SNMAC, Standing Nursing and Midwifery Advisory Committee (2001b) *Practice guidance: principles standards and indicators. Caring for older people: a nursing priority*. London: Department of Health.

Tromp AM, Pluijm SM, Smit JH, Deeg DJ, Bouter LM, Lips P (2001) Fall-risk screening test: a prospective study on predictors for falls in community – dwelling elders. *J Clin Epidemiol* 54: 837–844.

Wyatt J, Illingworth RN, Clancy MJ, Robertson CE (1999) *Oxford handbook of accident and emergency medicine*. Oxford: Oxford University Press.

6 | Mental health

Elizabeth Whelan

Patients with mental health disorders can pose some of the greatest challenges for emergency nurses. They have emotional, cognitive and behavioural needs influenced by culture and social stigma and may require psychological, social and medical interventions. Attendees with mental health problems only constitute up to 5% of patients attending Emergency Departments, while another 20–30% of attendees will have significant mental health problems co-existing with a physical disorder (DoH 1999). As with other patient groups the reasons for attendance vary from an acute event to requesting medication and the choice of the emergency service is dictated by its 24-h availability and its perceived ability to access the specialist provider. This chapter presents a structured approach to triage, assessment and diagnosis of patients with mental health disorders. Detailed guidance on patient management is provided in the form of care plans.

INTRODUCTION

Mentally ill patients are often professed to be unwelcome in the Emergency Department. This can be exacerbated by vagueness of presentation, appearing non-urgent – tiredness, worry and sleepless nights and their perceived lack of amenability to ABC algorithms (Wyatt et al 1999) and integrated care pathways. But failure to recognize or ensure follow-up for a mental health disorder denies the patient an opportunity for effective treatment. It is a missed opportunity to positively affect the quality of life for both them and their families (Warncken and Dolan 2000).

DIAGNOSIS OF MENTAL HEALTH DISORDERS

The most common aid to diagnosis is the International Classification of Diseases (ICD 10) (see Table 6.1).

Efforts have been made to create a hierarchy of symptoms (see Figure 6.1) with organic disorders at the top and personality disorders at the bottom (Davies 1997). A mental health problem is likely to show features of the category below it in the hierarchy but unlikely to show features of the disorders above it.

While this hierarchy is invaluable in gaining insight and understanding of disorders, care must be taken to consider co-morbidity of a physical disease with a psychiatric disorder or the co-existence of more than one psychiatric disorder.

TRIAGE

The purpose of the mental health triage assessment is to

- obtain a clear account of the patient's current problems,
- assess the nature and severity of the patient's current psychological and physical problems,
- assess treatment acuity,
- assess the patient's risk of harm to self or others,
- assess risk of absconding.

Currently no clear triage guidelines for prioritization of patients with mental health problems exist, so

Mental health

Table 6.1
International classification of diseases (ICD 10)

Category	Examples	Basic characteristics	Common presentations
Organic disorders	Dementia, delirium	Impaired memory, "organic" cause	Forgetfulness, confusion
Psychotic disorders	Schizophrenia, bipolar disorder	Delusions, hallucinations	Bizarre ideas, odd behaviour
Neurosis	Anxiety disorders, hypochondrias	Emotional disturbance	Worried, tired, physical complaints
Mood, stress related disorders	Depression, phobic disorder	Low mood, loss of pleasure	Tearful, fed up, physical complaints
Psychoactive substance use	Alcohol, opiate dependence, tobacco use	Psychological or physical effects of the substance	Addiction, withdrawal, depression
Personality disorder	Dissocial, paranoid	Dysfunctional personality traits	Exacerbation of traits when stressed

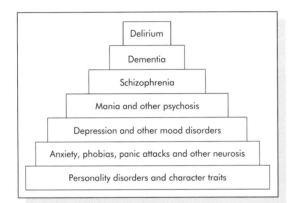

Figure 6.1 Hierarchy of mental health symptoms

local procedures must ensure that

- physical problems are not under triaged because of co-existing psychological problems,
- mini risk assessment is clearly recorded (see Table 6.2),
- the problem with the most immediate prioritization takes precedence.

Tables 6.2–6.4 (pp. 93–4) present three approaches to prioritizing the management of patients with mental health problems.

It must not be forgotten that chronic illnesses such as diabetes, alcoholism and injuries can affect neurological and mental status. Further examples can be found in Table 6.5 (p. 94).

DEPARTMENTAL ASSESSMENT

In order to devise a plan of care it is essential to expand on the triage assessment. Questions to be more fully answered include (South Eastern Sydney AHS 1998):

- Is the patient in distress?
- Is their condition likely to deteriorate?
- Are they physically ill?
- Are they able to co-operate with the assessment process?
- Is their behaviour likely to be unpredictable?
- Are they at risk?
- Are they likely to abscond?
- Is there a supportive person with them?
- What level of supervision will they require?

PSYCHOLOGICAL ASSESSMENT

In the absence of cognitive, emotional or behavioural problems a mini mental health assessment should still be completed. From *Lecture notes on psychiatry* (Harrison et al 1998) to the *Oxford handbook of Emergency Department medicine* (Wyatt et al 1999) the same fundamental principles form the core elements of a mini mental health assessment (**ABCDE** and **PREP**) (Whelan 2002):

- **A**ppearance,
- **B**ehaviour,

Table 6.2
Mini risk assessment

Problem	Immediate: priority 1 (P1)	<10 min: priority 2 (P2)	<60 min: priority 3 (P3)	<120 min: priority 4 (P4)	<240 min: priority 5 (P5)
Aggression violence	Actual violence – definite danger to self/others Severe distress	Aggressive – threats severe behavioural disturbance Severe distress	Frightened, impulsive, may be unpredictable Moderate behavioural disturbance	Mild distress Low danger to self or others	No danger to self or other No behavioural disturbance
Deliberate self-harm (DHS)	High suicide risk – brought in by others Effects of drug overdose Effects of gas Effects of hanging	High suicide – tries to leave Effects of drug overdose Deep lacerations	Moderate suicide risk But feels in control Mild distress	Low suicide risk Feels in control Anxious	No acute distress
Absconding	Attempts to abscond with physical aggression	Attempts to abscond but no physical aggression	Threats to abscond but no action taken	Low risk of absconding	Prepared to wait

Table 6.3
Potential mental health triage

Problem	Immediate: P1	<10 min: P2	<60 min: P3	<120 min: P4	<240 min: P5
Anxiety/ neurosis	Violence towards self/others, acute chaotic behaviour	Acute distress Requires assessment of acute medical problems	Moderate distress Threats to abscond	Mild symptoms of panic but feels in control	Medication request
Depression	DSH with acute medical problems	DSH with high suicidal intent Hostility towards self/others	History of alcohol withdrawal and fits since last drink	Depressed with no suicidal intent	Mild symptoms of depression and willing to wait
Psychosis	Acute behavioural problems with aggression/ violence	Clouding of consciousness with hostility, DSH	Hallucinations delusions with suicidal intent	Hallucinations No indications of risk to self/others	Long-term problems with no acute symptoms

- Cognitive ability and communication,
- Disposition,
- Emotional stability (see p. 95),

and

- Presenting problem and insight,
- Risk factors,
- Environment,
- Psychiatric history (see p. 95).

During the assessment the nurse needs to help the patient focus on the current problems while encouraging them to answer the question in their own words but not allowing them to ramble. If information needs

Table 6.4
Physical problems (as per local guidelines or Manchester triage) (Hammersmith Hospital NHS Trust 2000)

Problem	Immediate: P1	<10 min: P2	<60 min: P3	<120 min: P4	<240 min: P5
Self-inflicted wounds	Penetrating injury to chest or abdomen, pelvic area Gunshot/blast injuries Impaired circulation	Severe bleeding ++ uncontrolled by pressure dressing RR < 24, PR < 100	Bleeding ++ controlled by pressure dressing Joint penetration	Wound under 12 h old needing wound closure Grossly infected Foreign bodies	Over 12 h old Slight injuries Foreign body in situ over 12 h
Chest pain (acute anxiety, somatic disorder)	Severe pain central with radiation Shocked, grey, clammy	Sudden onset Known cardiac problems with risk factors All chest pain where a cardiac cause cannot be excluded		Associated with respiratory problems Productive cough Associated with rib injury	Long standing No acute problems
Fits (alcohol related)	Status epilepticus Current fitting Hypoglycaemia	Fitting more than two per hour Altered conscious level	Post-fit Confusion Drowsy, signs and symptoms of withdrawal	Post-ictal with no symptoms Has stopped drinking Anxiety	Requesting help, willing to wait, no withdrawal symptoms

Table 6.5
Effects of chronic illness on neurological and mental functioning (Good and Nelson 1986)

Hyperthyroidism	Hyperactivity, pressured speech, and mimic "mania"; irritability, impulsiveness
Hypothyroidism	Depression, withdrawal, apathy
Antihypertensives (Aldomet)	Depression
Severe blood loss	Delirium (due to poor brain perfusion)
Cimetidine	Toxic psychosis
Pancreatic carcinoma Lung cancer Pheochromocytomas	Depression Progressive dementia Anxiety or manic attacks
Temporal lobe epilepsy	Schizophrenia or manic like behaviour
Hypokalemia	Anxiety, depression
Alcohol abuse Alcohol withdrawal	Major personality changes Delirium; hallucinations, acute anxiety
Cocaine Amphetamines	Transient – grandiosity Depression, transient paranoid psychosis

Elizabeth Whelan

Mini mental health assessment

Appearance: consider – clothing, neglect, nutrition, and body language, facial expression, suggestions of drug or alcohol abuse.

Behaviour: consider – unusual movements, psychomotor activity, and reaction to the assessment.

Communication and cognitive ability: consider:

- *Communication* – speech, content, non-verbal communication.
- *Cognitive ability* – mini mental state examination (see Figure 6.2, p. 96).

NB: Remember to consider language barriers and cultural influences.

Disposition: consider – mood (subjective, objective), frame of mind, feelings.

Emotional stability: consider – thought process, content, paranoia/delusions, perceptual distortions and hallucinations.

and

Presenting problem and insight:

- *Presenting problem* – nature and length of episode, main problem, other problems, any current physical illness, recent trauma, affect on daily lives?
- *Insight* – assess the understanding of the present difficulties and do they correctly identify the relevance of their symptoms?

Risk assessment: consider risk to the following:

- Health/well being through poor nutrition, self-neglect, vulnerability to assault, exploitation, sexual exploitation, exhaustion or dehydration.
- Patient's safety through suicide, deliberate self-harm or chaotic behaviour.
- Others such as family, children (through neglect), a newborn baby and staff (Atakan 1997).
- A detailed risk assessment (risk factors or assessment tools) (Harrison et al 1998) is for all patients with:
  - expressed suicidal intentions (assessment tools are presented in Figure 6.3, p. 97)
  - history of mood disorder, psychosis or substance abuse (see Figure 6.4, p. 97)
  - history of self-harm or violence.

Environment: consider – personal and social history: Does the patient live alone? Do they have support or come from a chaotic, disruptive environment? What is their employment status, housing status? Do they have any financial difficulties? Is there a family history of mental health problems?

Past psychiatric history: consider – previous psychiatric episodes? Current treatment/medication, mental state between episodes – completely well or maintained on therapy?

to be elicited from accompanying friends and relatives it must be documented.

PHYSICAL ASSESSMENT

Physical examination is important, as there may be a co-existing physical and mental health problem. It is necessary to rule out or confirm organic causes of presenting symptoms. The literature recommends no standard approach to examination for patients with mental health problems, varying from a brief examination of all systems to examination of relevant systems as indicated by current symptoms, current medication and past medical history.

Any acute medical problems identified should be addressed immediately and vital signs, blood sugar and head to toe observation for injury (signs of self-harm, track marks) recorded. Tests and investigations that are frequently indicated include – ECG, CT scans, baseline blood screen and tests for endocrine abnormalities.

Mental health

Assess	Method	Score
Orientation for time	Day, date, month, season, year	1 point each
Orientation for place	Country, county, city/town, hospital, name of the ward	1 point each
Learning of new information	Name three unrelated objects (clock, umbrella, carrot) Patient must learn all three objects	1 point each – at first attempt only
Attention and concentration	Spell "world" backwards	1 point each letter in the correct order
Short term memory	"Name the three items that we named a few minutes ago"	1 point each
Language	Point to a pen and wristwatch and ask the patient to name them	2 points
	Repeat the phrase "no ifs, ands or buts"	1 point
	Tell the patient to follow these instructions "take this piece of paper in your right hand, fold it in half and put it on the floor"	1 point for each part
	Read and obey: show the patient a piece of paper with the phrase "close your eyes" written on it and ask them to follow the instructions	1 point
	Ask the patient to write a short sentence	1 point – if it makes sense
	Ask the patient to copy a diagram – two five sided shapes which are intersecting	1 point

(Based on Wyatt et al 1999; Seidal et al 1995)
A score of 20 or less out of the 30 is suggestive of confusion or impaired communication.

Figure 6.2 The mini mental state examination

PLANNING CARE

The plan of care requires a range of psychological, pharmacological or social options dictated by the medical and/or mental health assessment, diagnosis, risk assessment and stage of the illness. The principles are defined simply by Harrison et al (1998) as follows:

- Is treatment required?
- How urgent is the problem?
- Where should the treatment take place and who should provide it?
- What management is indicated?

Any attendance at Emergency Department is filled with anxiety provoking stimuli; nurses can help reduce this by following these guidelines (Hudak and Gallo 1994):

- Providing order so the patient can prepare for what is to happen
- Inform them what is about to happen so they can muster their coping mechanism
- Allowing choice when possible to increase a sense of control
- Include the patient in decisions
- Providing information and explanation.

This must be built into the individual care plans incorporating triage priority, mini mental health assessment, intervention and risk assessment. Common presentations to the Emergency Department include:

- psychosis,
- depression,

Assessment tool	Suicide risk
Beck depression inventory: patient picks the best answer	3 = I would kill myself if I had the chance 2 = I have definite plans about committing suicide 1 = I feel I would be better off dead 0 = I do not have any thoughts of harming myself
Hamilton depression rating scale: rater selects best answer	0 = Thoughts of suicide absent 1 = Feels life is not worth living 2 = Wishes he or she were dead or any thoughts of possible death to self 3 = Suicide ideas or gesture 4 = Attempts at suicide (and serious attempt rates 4)
Symptom checklist: patient rates on five-point scale from not at all to extremely	How much were you bothered by: Thoughts of ending your life Thoughts of death or dying
Sad persons scale <3 low risk 3–6 medium risk >6 high risk	S sex (female = 0, male = 1) A age (<19 or >45 = 1, otherwise 0) D depression/hopelessness = 1 P previous attempts score = 1 E excessive alcohol/drug use = 1 R rational thinking loss (psychotic or organic illness) score 1 S separated, widowed, divorced = 1 O organized or serious attempt = 1 N no social support score = 1 S stated future intent score = 1

(Based on Priory.com 2000; Paterson et al 1983)

Figure 6.3 Suicide risk assessment tools

If the patient answers "yes" to three or more questions there is likely to be problem: for example, with alcohol the likelihood is 250 : 1
(Harrison et al 1998)

If the patient admits to drinking alcohol then the CAGE question should be asked:

■ Have you ever thought you should **C**ut down on your drinking?
■ Have people ever **A**nnoyed you by criticizing your drinking?
■ Have you ever felt **G**uilty about your drinking?
■ Have you ever had an **E**ye-opener (drink) first thing in the morning?

Figure 6.4 Assessing alcohol or drug use using CAGE (Mayfield et al 1974)

■ anxiety/neurosis,
■ deliberate self-harm.

Care plans for these four aspects of mental health care are presented on the next four pages (98–101).

THE MENTAL HEALTH ACT (1983)

While most treatment for a mental disorder is undertaken voluntarily both in the community and hospital, occasionally compulsory treatment is required. Compulsory admission is only considered if all attempts at persuasion to be admitted voluntarily have failed. The reasons for admission must comply with the Mental Health Act (MHA). These include a mental disorder so severe as to warrant treatment in hospital for the patient's health, safety and/or the protection of others. The most commonly used sections of the MHA are identified in Table 6.6 (p. 102).

Care Plan 1 Psychosis

History: Presenting problem: delusions (victim of a conspiracy), bizarre behaviour amphetamine use, self-neglect, refuses help, talking to themselves, auditory or visual hallucinations, distressed, side effects of medication. **Differential diagnosis:** schizophrenia, psychosis in depression or mania, puerperal psychosis, organic or drug induced psychosis, cerebral tumour, alcohol abuse, encephalitis, head injury.

Mental health assessment: Mini mental health assessment – A – bizarre (to prevent thought extraction), poor hygiene? B – Stupor? Disorganized, C – thought salad, thought insertion by others? Being read by others? Broadcasting? D – flattened effect? Inappropriate effect? **Insight** – is able to distinguish reality from own perceptions? **Mental state examination** – score. **Physical examination:** signs of poor nutrition, weight loss, organic causes – drug induced states, Symptoms of distress – hyperventilation (anxiety) raised P & BP (agitated behaviour) which may mask physical disorders (infections, endocrine).

Interventions: If somatic symptoms – normal range of laboratory tests, vital signs, blood sugar, others as indicated by physical examination – CT scan.

Risk Assessment: Violence and aggression own health (self-neglect), others (auditory commands, neglect children as a result of the carers erratic behaviour).

Triage rating: 1
Risk: high
Plan of care:
- Treat with empathy
- Treat acute medical problems
- Treat acute extra-pyramidal side effects
- Continuous observation of mental and physical state
- Monitor as dictated by risk of absconding, violence
- Refer to psychiatric liaison team

Evaluation:
- Prompt action taken
- Appropriate persons informed
- Patient distress reduced
- Admit under appropriate team

Triage rating: 2
Risk: high to medium
Plan of care:
- Treat with empathy, reduce external stimuli
- Listen to delusions seriously but do not collude
- Assess acuity of medical problems and treat.
- Refer to psychiatric liaison team
- Monitor closely
- Anti-psychotic drugs to alleviate acute symptoms
- Support patient through admission

Evaluation:
- Patient distress reduced
- Admit under appropriate specialist team

Triage rating: 3
Risk: Medium
Plan of care:
- Sit with patient if time available and offer emotional support
- If hallucinating be factual and professional
- Check regularly for deterioration in mental status
- Keep informed of departmental routine
- Refer to psychiatric liaison team
- Check compliance with depot injections if poor insight

Evaluation:
- Patient anxiety minimized
- Appropriate decisions made
- Positive out come achieved

Triage rating: 4
Risk: low
Plan of care:
- Check regularly
- Reassure that help is available, ensure that the patient is not provoked by others
- Assess knowledge deficit
- Health care team to determine if discharge appropriate
- Medication as prescribed
- Encourage to adhere to medication

Evaluation:
- Deterioration limited
- Ensure supportive environment and community team informed
- Patient is aware where to access support in a crisis

Triage rating: 5
Risk: none
Plan of care:
- Safe and observable area
- Monitor regularly
- Monitor for extra-pyramidal effects of long-term medication
- Keep patient informed of waiting times
- Access to food/drinks

Evaluation:
- Reduced anxiety
- Appropriate discharge
- Supportive environment in place either family or community care
- Community team informed
- Patient is fully informed and concurs

References: Lemma 1996; Harrison et al 1998; Turner 1998; Wyatt et al 1998; Warncken and Dolan 2000; Polli and Lazear 2000.

Elizabeth Whelan

Care Plan 2 Depression

History: Presenting problem: "I've lost my appetite, can't sleep" tiredness, suicidal ideation, aches and pains, inability to cope, tearful,
Risk Factors: drugs, family death, divorce, loneliness, holiday, child birth, chronic illness/pain, job loss.

Mental health assessment: Mini mental health assessment – A – self-neglect? B – retardation in movement? Slow? Stupor? Disturbed? C – retardation of speech, withdrawn? D – mood, low, hopelessness? **Insight** – the patient's understanding of current problems. **Mental state examination:** score (poor concentration). **Physical examination:** signs of poor nutrition, weight loss, constipation, organic cause – hypothyroidism, antihypertensives, other organic causes.

Interventions if somatic symptoms – ECG, normal range of laboratory tests, liver, thyroid function tests, vital signs, blood sugar.

Risk Assessment: Own health (stops eating drinking, self-neglect), others (neglect children, behavioural changes).

Triage rating: 1
Risk: high: high suicide risk, risk of aggression, poor nutritional state
Plan of care:
- Treat with empathy understanding
- Treat acute medical problems
- Continuous 1:1 nursing
- Monitor mental and physical state all times for deterioration
Evaluation:
- Prompt action taken
- Appropriate persons informed
- Admit under appropriate specialist team

Triage rating: 2
Risk: high to medium
Plan of care:
- Treat with empathy and understanding
- Assess acuity of medical problems and treat accordingly.
- Refer to psychiatric liaison team
- Suicide assessment
- Monitor closely
- Offer support and reassurance
Evaluation:
- Prompt action taken
- Appropriate persons informed
- Admit under appropriate specialist team

Triage rating: 3
Risk: medium
Plan of care:
- Sit with patient if time available and offer emotional support
- Check regularly for deterioration in mental status
- Keep informed of departmental routine
- Allow time for alcohol effects to subside provided there is no risk
- Refer to psychiatric liaison team
- Support patient through admission if required due to severity and risk
Evaluation:
- Appropriate decisions made
- Positive outcome achieved

Triage rating: 4
Risk: low
Plan of care:
- Check regularly
- Assess knowledge deficit
- Health care team to determine if discharge appropriate
- Medication as prescribed
- Counselling organized if appropriate
- Consider Psychiatric outpatients appointment
Evaluation:
- If discharged check that a supportive environment is in place
- Community team informed
- Patient is fully informed and concurs

Triage rating: 5
Risk: none
Plan of care:
- Safe and observable area
- Monitor regularly
- Keep patient informed of waiting times
- Access to food/drinks
Evaluation:
- Appropriate discharge
- Supportive environment in place
- Community team informed
- Patient is fully informed and concurs

References: Harrison et al 1998; Wyatt et al 1999; Kumar and Clark 2000.

Mental health

Care Plan 3 Anxiety/Neurosis

History: Presenting problem: difficulty in breathing, flushed, hyperventilation, dizziness, insomnia, palpitations sweating, trigger (shock, crowd) family history, feeling of impending doom. **Differential diagnosis:** acute anxiety, panic disorders, phobias, depression, obsessive compulsive disorder, somatic disorder.

Mental health assessment: Mini mental health assessment – B – seeks re-assurance, chaotic, restless, agitated, withdrawn, terrified. C – increased tone, rate, uncommunitive, self-obsessed. D – detached, irritable, anxious? **Insight** – assess level, Mental State Examination: score (difficulty concentrating).
Physical examination: Respiratory (hyperventilation) tachycardia, rule out organic cause of signs and symptoms.

Interventions if somatic symptoms – vital signs, arterial blood gases (impaired gas exchange), ECG, CXR, others as indicated by physical examination.

Risk Assessment: violence, suicide, self-harm, self (disorganized, inability to make thoughtful judgements) chaotic behaviour.

Triage rating: 1
Risk: high of violence, suicide
Plan of care:
- Minimize extraneous stimulation
- Remove potential weapons
- Ensure support staff available including security, police
- Calm, conversational approach
- Restraint as temporary control method
- Continuous observation
Evaluation:
- Prompt action taken
- Appropriate persons informed
- Patient distress reduced

Triage rating: 2
Risk: high to medium
Plan of care:
- Treat acute medical problems
- Build trusting relationship
- Be calm and supportive, Reduce external stimuli
- Treat hyperventilation by rebreathing (assisting patient with problem solving activity) minor tranquillizer
- Explain all procedures in simple and consistent terms
- Suicide/self-harm risk assessment
- Monitor closely
- Refer to psychiatric liaison team? Admission
Evaluation:
- Patient distress reduced

Triage rating: 3
Risk: medium
Plan of care:
- Sit with patient if time available and offer emotional support
- Reduce environmental stimuli
- Assess acuity of medical problems and treat
- Assess knowledge deficit
- Encourage to begin problem solving process – such as devising coping strategies
- Refer to psychiatric liaison team – to determine if judgement is impaired
Evaluation:
- Deterioration limited
- Encouraged to problem solve
- Positive out come achieved

Triage rating: 4
Risk: low
Plan of care:
- Check regularly and keep informed
- Reassure that help is available
- Encourage to voice concerns and identify means of preventing recurrence
- Keep informed of departmental routine
- Encourage to adhere to medication
Evaluation:
- Patient anxiety reduced
- Ensure supportive environment and community team informed
- Patient is aware where to access support in a crisis

Triage rating: 5
Risk: none
Plan of care:
- Safe and observable area
- Monitor discreetly
- Encourage to discuss triggering factors
- Allow time to discuss worries and coping strategies
- Keep patient informed of waiting times
- Access to food/drinks
Evaluation:
- Reduced anxiety
- Appropriate discharge
- Supportive environment in place either family or community care
- GP/community team informed
- Patient is fully informed

References: Polli and Lazear 2000; Kumar and Clark 2000; South Eastern Sydney AHS 1998.

Elizabeth Whelan

Care Plan 4 Deliberate Self-harm

History: Presenting problem: where and how, precipitating circumstances, preparation, concealment, suicidal intent, accidental discovery or self-presentation, alcohol/drug misuse, domestic violence. **Risk factors:** single, separated, loss, male, elderly, social support, isolation, previous self-harm, suicide attempts, personality disorder, angry, depressed, alcohol, chronic medical problems, poor coping skills.

Mental health assessment: Mini mental health assessment – A – tearful, self-neglect, cuts on arms (previous self-harm) B – restless, agitated? C – unresponsive, threats of self-harm? D – angry? Depressed? Guilty? **Insight** – the patient's understanding of current problems. **Mental state examination:** score. **Physical examination:** dictated by method of self-harm – features of overdose, physical injuries, known physical illness.

Interventions: As indicated by injuries, drugs taken, physical examination – ECG, normal range of laboratory tests, paracetamol, salicylate levels, vital signs, X-ray.

Risk Assessment: To self, suicide risk score (see assessment tools), to others (aggression/violence if interferes in a suicide attempt, interferes when

Triage rating: 1
Risk: high
Plan of care:
- Treat with empathy understanding
- Treat acute medical problems (hanging, certain overdoses)
- Continuous 1 : 1 supervision or higher according to risk
- Risk assessments
- Restrain in extreme circumstances
- Admit under MHA if appropriate
Evaluation:
- Prompt action taken
- Admit under appropriate specialist team

Triage rating: 2
Risk: high to medium
Plan of care:
- Sit with patient if time allows, set regular observation times
- Encourage to talk and treat with empathy
- Assess acuity of medical problems and treat overdose (lacerations)
- Risk assessments
- Refer to psychiatric liaison team
Evaluation:
- Prompt action taken
- Appropriate persons informed
- Admit under appropriate specialist team

Triage rating: 3
Risk: medium
Plan of care:
- Monitor regularly until suicidal ideation minimized
- Offer emotional support
- Suicide risk assessment
- Allow time for alcohol effects to subside provided there is no risk
- Treat under lying mental illness
- Refer to psychiatric liaison team especially if psychotic symptoms
- Support patient through admission if required due to severity and risk
Evaluation:
- Appropriate decisions made
- Positive outcome achieved

Triage rating: 4
Risk: medium to low
Plan of care:
- Discreet observations
- Identify means of preventing recurrence
- Health care team to determine if discharge appropriate
- Medication as prescribed
- Counselling organized if appropriate
- Psychiatric outpatients appointment if probable mental illness
Evaluation:
- Support contacts available
- Community self-harm team is informed
- Patient is fully informed and concurs

Triage rating: 5
Risk: none
Plan of care:
- Safe and observable area
- Monitor regularly
- Provide opportunity to discuss problems
- Refer to social worker if problem social
- Keep patient informed of waiting times
- Access to food/drinks
- Inform GP
- Home with friend/family
Evaluation:
- Appropriate discharge
- Supportive environment in place
- Community self-harm team is informed
- Patient is fully informed

References: Jones 1996; Atakan and Davies 1997; Kumar and Clark 2000; South Eastern Sydney AHS 1998.

Table 6.6
Sections of the Mental Health Act (1983) commonly used in Emergency Departments (Jones and Morris 1992)

Section	Purpose	Requested by
2	Admission for assessment – required to prevent harm to self or others	Approved social worker (ASW) Approved doctor under Section 12 of the act
3	Admission for psychiatric treatment	ASW Approved doctor under Section 12 of the act
4	Emergency admission (approved psychiatrist not available)	ASW Doctor
5(2)	To stop an inpatient leaving the hospital – this does not allow treatment to be enforced	Responsible consultant or deputy (medical team responsible for patient) – then contact a psychiatrist
136	Allows police to take a person to a place of safety – if that person is behaving in a dangerous or bizarre manner in a public place and a psychiatric disorder is suspected	Police

In an acute emergency, detention or treatment can be given under common law when in the best interests of the patient (Barker 1998) though only what is considered reasonable (Harrison et al 1998). *The MHA only covers mental health disorders and cannot therefore be used to implement medical treatment.*

DOCUMENTATION

As a guide to future management and in order for any diagnosis reached to be set in context a succinct summary of the presentation must be recorded. This should include:

- Date and time of assessment, name of assessor
- Full details of any behavioural problems encountered and any action taken
- Details of psychiatric and physical assessments, include both positive and negative findings (Brown 1996)
- Source of information and relationship to patient
- Plan: treatment goals and/or reason for referral to any other agency
- Evaluation of any care given.

N.B. It is vital to remember that risk assessment is a dynamic process and assessment must be reviewed regularly as part of the plan of care.

DISCHARGE PLANNING

Discharge planning is vital to ensure the sharing of consistent information and the on-going management of the patient's care.

Ensure the patient and carers are aware of the following:
- Their diagnosis and any future care required
- Proposed time of discharge
- Medications: instructions for administration, side effects, where and when to get a follow-up prescription
- Where to attend in a crisis/who can be contacted, e.g. Samaritans
- Who has been informed – GP, CPN, community services.

References/Bibliography

Atakan Z, Davies T (1997) ABC of mental health: mental health emergencies. *Br Med J* 314(7096): 1740–1742.

Barker A (1998) Mental health and the law. *ABC of mental health*, Chapter 17. London: BMJ Books.

Brown AFT (1996) *Emergency medicine diagnosis and management*, 3rd ed. Melbourne: Butterworth Heinneman.

Davies T (1997) ABC of mental health: mental health assessment. *Br Med J* 314(7093): 1536–1539.

Department of Health (1999) *Mental health: national service frameworks*. London: Department of Health.

Good WV, Nelson JE (1986) *Psychiatry made ridiculously simple*, 3rd ed. Miami: MedMaster, Inc.

Hammersmith Hospitals NHS Trust (2000) *Triage package*. Hammersmith Hospitals NHS Trust, unpublished.

Harrison P, Geddes J, Sharpe M (1998) *Lecture notes on psychiatry*, 8th ed. Oxford: Blackwell Science Ltd.

Hudak CM, Gallo BM, eds (1994) *Critical care nursing: a holistic approach*, 6th ed. Philadelphia: J.B. Lippincott Company.

Jones L (1996) Assessing suicide risk in A&E. *Emergen Nurs* 2(4): 7–9.

Jones MA, Morris AE (1992) *Blackstone's statutes on medical law*. London: Blackstone Press Limited.

Kumar P, Clark M, eds (2000) *Acute general medicine*. Oxford: Butterworth Heinemann.

Lemma A (1996) *Introduction to psychopathology*. London: Sage Publications Ltd.

Manchester Triage Group (1997) *Emergency triage*. London: BMJ Publishing Group.

Mason T, Chandley M (1999) *Managing violence and aggression*. Edinburgh: Churchill Livingstone.

Mayfield D, McLeod G, Hall P (1974). The CAGE questionnaire: validation of a new alcoholism screening instrument. *Amer J Psychiat* 131: 1121–1123.

Paterson WM, Dohn HH, Bird J, Patterson GA (1983) 'Evaluation of suicidal patients: the SAD PERSON Scale' *Psychosomatics* 24(4): 343–349.

Polli GE, Lazear SE (2000) Mental health emergencies. *Emergency nursing core curriculum/emergency nurses association*, 5th ed. Chapter 10. Philadelphia: WB Saunders Company.

Priory.com (2000) The assessment of risk. http://www.priory.com/psych/risk.htm, 13/11/2000.

Seidal HM, Ball JW, Dains JE, Benedict GW (1995) *Physical examination handbook*. St. Louis: Mosby.

South Eastern Sydney Area Health Service (1998) *Training manual for non-mental health trained staff to work with mental health patients in hospital emergency departments*. Area Mental Health Program, South Eastern Sydney Area Health Service, unpublished.

Turner T (1998) Schizophrenia. *ABC of mental health*, Chapter 8. London: BMJ Books.

Warncken B, Dolan B (2000) Psychiatric emergencies. *Accident and emergency theory into practice*, Chapter 10. London: Bailliere Tindall, Royal College of Nursing.

Whelan E (2002) Vulnerable groups. *Medical assessment units*, Chapter 11. London: Whurr Publishers.

Wyatt JP, Illingworth RN, Clancy MJ, Munro PT, Robertson CE (1999) *Oxford handbook of accident and emergency medicine*. Oxford: Oxford University Press.

Elizabeth Whelan

7 | Major trauma management

Maureen O'Reilly

Much attention has been focused on trauma over the past two decades, with the emphasis on improving our understanding of physiological processes and achieving better outcomes for patients. This activity is highlighted in the number of systems now available for faster assessment of patients and rapid classification of trauma injuries. This approach has resulted in a greatly improved understanding of how to optimize management of the trauma patient and is reflected in this chapter. The chapter focuses on the management of trauma in adult patients. Assessment and interventions may take place in the pre-hospital setting or the Emergency Department, depending on local service configuration.

EPIDEMIOLOGY OF TRAUMA

Trauma is a term used to describe the variety of injuries, and is an international problem. It has been associated with several terms: accident, accidental injury, casualty, shock, injury. It is the leading cause of death in the population of between 1 and 45 years of age and the fourth cause of death across all ages groups, preceded by heart disease, cancer and strokes. Hence, reduction in trauma morbidity and mortality is an international goal. Death is known to occur at three key intervals/peaks – *first*: within minutes of the injury, *second*: within 2 h after injury, and *third*: weeks after the incident often due to complications.

In the past 60 years, health care providers, politicians and the public sector have recognized the need to address the rising accident rates and costs to the individual and society. Consequently, there has been an increase in research and community based projects to educate the public in safety/prevention, first aid and immediate life support.

MECHANISMS OF INJURY/ BIOMECHANICS

Mechanisms of injury are based on *kinematics*, which is the process of evaluating the probability of injuries based on

- forces and motion involved in the trauma;
- accident information gleaned at the time of initial assessment;
- a high index of suspicion by the practitioner for injuries;

and on *principles of physics*. Newton's first law of motion is most frequently cited:

"a body at rest will remain at rest, and a body in motion will remain in motion until acted on by an outside force".

Hence, the extent of injury is based on two factors:

1 the amount/magnitude of energy, speed or velocity;
2 the duration of impact.

The human body will absorb energy, and injury will occur when the tissue limits fail.

The factors influencing injury are therefore summarized as

- *tensile strength* – the amount of tension a tissue can withstand and the ability to resist stretching forces;

- *elasticity* – ability to resume the original size and shape after being stretched;
- *compressive strength* – ability to resist squeezing forces or inward pressure;
- *acceleration* – change in rate or speed of a moving body;
- *deceleration* – decrease in velocity of a moving object;
- *shearing force* – occur across a plane with structures slipping relative to each other.

Hence information gained at the scene of the incident is invaluable when treating the patient in the Emergency Department.

The type of injury that results can be identified as

1 *Non-penetrating/blunt* – an injury with no communication to the outside environment is potentially life threatening as the extent of injury is less obvious, often making diagnosis more difficult. The forces are acceleration, deceleration, compression. The common causes are motor vehicle crashes, falls, assaults and contact sports.
2 *Penetrating injuries* – are caused when an outside or foreign object is set into motion;

the extent of the injury is dependent upon knowing
- the type and characteristic of object/agent;
- energy dissipation (low velocity or high velocity);
- tissue characteristics (dense/loose);
- distance from the weapon to individual target.

The common causes are stab wounds, impalements, gunshot wounds.
3 *Other injuries* – explosive blasts occur when detonated explosives are converted to large volumes of gases, causing fragments to become high-velocity missiles, and the blast shock wave to cause damage at air-tissue contacts.

The utilization of a trauma scoring system can be of benefit both for individual patient care and wider service development at local and national level. Some examples of the uses of scoring systems are highlighted in Figure 7.1.

INITIAL PATIENT ASSESSMENT

The initial assessment is composed of two parts – the primary and secondary surveys. The goal of the

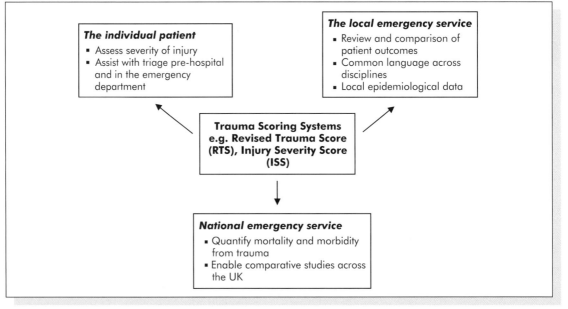

Figure 7.1 Uses of scoring system data

Maureen O'Reilly

primary survey is to simultaneously identify and intervene in life-threatening injuries. The secondary survey is begun after completing the primary survey, ensuring resuscitation efforts are proceeding correctly and comprises a complete head-to-toe assessment. It is imperative to remember the cervical spine must be stabilized/immobilized during the primary survey and airway assessment stage. Cervical immobilization may be effectively completed using manual-in-line stabilization, cervical collar (rigid), sandbags, taping or other specialized immobilization devices.

PRIMARY SURVEY

A. Airway

Ensure that
   the airway is patent;
   speech/sounds age appropriate are present;
   the cervical spine is immobilized if not
      yet done;
   there is no visible foreign material in the upper
      airway: tongue, secretions, food, vomit, blood,
      teeth/dental plate, other debris.

Look for
   airway/facial/inhalation injury
   obstructive signs:
      snoring – below pharynx;
      crowing – laryngeal spasm;
      gurgling – foreign body;
      wheezing – bronchospasm.

Intervention may include one or more of the following:
   chinlift/jaw thrust, *never hyper-extend
      the neck*;
   suction to clear the airway;
   airway adjuncts;
      nasopharyngeal or oropharyngeal
         airway;
      orotracheal/nasotracheal intubation;
      oesophageal obturator airway;
      laryngeal mask airway;
      needle cricothyroidotomy;
      surgical cricothyroidotomy;
      tracheotomy
      hyperoxygenate 100% (×30 min);

B. Breathing

Assess initially, reassess every 15 min
Ensure that
   respirations are spontaneous and unlaboured;
   chest expansion is equal and bilateral/chest rise
      and fall is symmetrical;
   breath sounds are present bilaterally.

Look for
   tachypnoea (moderate ↑ 20; severe ↑ 30);
   apnoea;
   respiratory rate <10 or >24/min (adult)
      deviations appropriate for paediatric age;
   weak, shallow, respirations;
   diminished or absent breath sounds;
   paradoxical respirations;
   unequal pulmonary exhalation;
   cyanosis;
   tracheal deviation;
   distended neck veins;
   anxious, restless, confused, stuporous, comatose
      external signs of trauma;
   open chest wound;
   subcutaneous emphysema.

Worry about and simultaneously treat:
   tension pneumothorax;
   large flail segment, pulmonary contusion;
   open pneumothorax;
   massive haemothorax;

Intervention may include one or more of the following:
   provide oxygenation;
   needle thoracotomy;
   chest occlusive dressing;
   chest tubes/auto-transfusion.

C. Circulation

Assess initially, reassess every 15 min.
Ensure that
   the patient is conscious and alert;
   absence of obvious uncontrolled external
      bleeding;
   full, regular peripheral pulses (bilateral absence
      of radial pulses indicates
      systolic blood pressure (SBP) <80 mmHg;
      loss of femoral pulse <70 mmHg;
      loss of carotid pulse <60 mmHg)
   heart sounds appropriate.

Look for
   altered mental state/level of consciousness;
   skin pale, cool, diaphoretic;
   capillary refill >3 s;
   in the adult patient, heart rate < 50 or >120;
   thready, irregular central pulse, not able to obtain
    at more than one site;
   Becks Triad – systolic hypotension ↓ and
    pressure and neck veins muffled HS elevated
    central venous pressure (CVP);
   SBP < 90 mmHg;
   external exsanguinating haemorrhage.

Worry about and simultaneously treat
   fluid volume deficit;
   exsanguinating external haemorrhage;
   pericardial tamponade.

Classifications of haemorrhage

Class I: Loss – 15% circulating volume (750 ml)
Signs and symptoms
   none to minimal (auto-transfusion occurring),
   Slight anxiety,
   Heart rate < 100, SBP – normal,
   Pulse pressure normal/slightly↑
   Respiratory rate 14–20/min
   Cap refill within 2 s
   Cool skin urine output > 30 ml/h
   (10% loss arterial pressure ↓ 7%,
    cardiac output ↓ 20%)
   Fluids – crystalloids

Class II: Loss – 20–25% volume (1000–1500 ml)
Signs and symptoms
   Heart rate > 100, SBP ↓, Diastolic blood
    pressure (DBP) ↑, ↓ pulse
   Pressure delay in capillary refill, Pale cool skin
   (20% loss arterial pressure ↓ 15%,
    cardiac output ↓ 40%)
   Urine output 20–30 ml/h
   Fluids – crystalloids

Class III: Loss – 30–40% volume (1500–2000 ml)
Signs and symptoms
   ↑ Heart rate, ↓ blood pressure,
    ↓ pulse pressure, ↑↑ thirst
   Respiratory rate 30→40/min
   Agitated, ↓ clarity
   Cool moist skin

   Urine output 5–15 ml/h
   Fluids – replace crystalloids 3:1,
    blood replacement

Class IV: Loss – >50% volume (200–500 ml)
Signs and symptoms
   Dilated pupils, loss of consciousness (LOC),
   Absent/bare vital signs heart rate > 140,
    respiratory rate > 35
   Oliguria
   Cold, cyanotic, mottled skin
   Fluids – blood replacement

D. Debilitation

Brief neuro/level of consciousness assessment
Glasgow Coma Scale
Pupillary response.

E. Exposure

Completely undress to facilitate examination and
re-evaluation
Keep patient warm.

F. Full vital signs

Blood pressure, pulse, respiratory rate
Temperature
Cardiac monitoring.

SECONDARY SURVEY

The purpose is to note and treat other injuries in a
systematic head to toe approach.

   *Examine each area of the body for old and new signs
of injury: contusions, abrasions, lacerations, swelling,
ecchymosis (bruising), entry/exit wounds, impaled objects,
scars.*

   In addition check the following:

Head

■ Check scalp, eyes and eyelids, palpate facial
  prominences
■ Examine the skull for depressions, deformities,
  penetrating wounds
■ Evaluate for
  – Basilar skull fracture
  – Battle's sign
  – Raccoon's eyes – periorbital ecchymosis

- Examine for (serous) otorrhoea, rhinorrhoea, or blood from nares/ear canal
- Examine mouth for blood, vomit, dental plates/teeth, debris, inhalation burns.

Neck

- Palpate for point tenderness over cervical spine area
- Evaluate for distended or flat jugular veins
- Palpate for tracheal deviation, tenderness, subcutaneous emphysema
- Note changes in voice/presence of hoarseness.

Chest

- Examine for penetrating wounds, sucking sounds
- Palpate clavicles, rib cage, sternum
- Auscultate bilateral breath sounds, heart sounds
- Inspect for symmetrical chest expansion
- Identify paradoxical breathing
- Evaluate cardiac rhythm on monitor.

Abdomen

- Auscultate for bowel sounds
- Palpate light and deep, assess for the presence of tenderness, guarding, rigidity.

Pelvis

- Gently compress iliac crests.

Genital area

- Inspect for obvious injuries
- Note presence of blood at urinary meatus
- Inspect labia/scrotal/penile area for haematoma
- Assist with rectal examination.

Extremities

- Inspect for swelling, deformity, dislocation, protrusion of bones, bleeding, obvious fractures;
- Palpate for point tenderness at suspected fracture sites, crepitus
- Assess neurovascular-sensation and pulses present and equal bilaterally
- Look for the 5 p's indicating vascular occlusion:

P Pain
Pallor
Pulses
Paraesthesia
Paralysis

Back

- The patient is carefully log rolled to one side, maintaining spinal alignment
- Palpate entire spinal/vertebral length for deformities, point tenderness (especially thoracic and lumbar areas)
- Assist in assessment of rectal tone.

Neuro

- Re-evaluate LOC/Glasgow Coma Scale, presence of sensory/motor loss and pupil assessment for potential raised intracranial pressure.

Any localized injury will necessitate more focused examination and diagnostic studies.

Additional data gathered during the secondary survey includes:

Subjective data collection

- The chief complaint
- Treatment received prior to arrival
- Known allergies
- Tetanus immunization status
- Current medical status: previous medical conditions and surgical interventions
- Current medications (prescribed, over the counter products used, herbal/alternative therapies)
- Gynaecological history – Last menstrual period, gestation, pregnancies, miscarriages, abortions.

General overview

- Continuing vital sign assessment
- General appearance
- Characteristic/unusual odours – alcohol, gasoline, chemicals, faeces, urine.

Shock

Shock is a clinical syndrome characterized by lack of tissue perfusion needed to meet the oxygen and nutritional needs of the cell.

Cardiogenic shock includes both coronary (myocardial infarction, coronary artery disease) and non-coronary causes (valvular disorders, cardiomyopathies, cardiac tamponade and arrhythmias).

Distributive vasogenic types include the neurogenic, septic and anaphylactic forms. Adequate blood supply can be diminished in the vascular bed due to decreased volume/fluid loss (hypovolaemic or haemorrhagic shock), increased peripheral vasodilation or changes in vascular resistance (neurogenic, septic or anaphylactic shock) or inadequate pumping ability of the heart (both forms of cardiogenic shock).

The overall effect is such that the diminished blood flow decreases venous return to the heart, which in turn reduces cardiac output causing a low volume state, decreasing delivery of oxygen and nutrients to the cell for consumption.

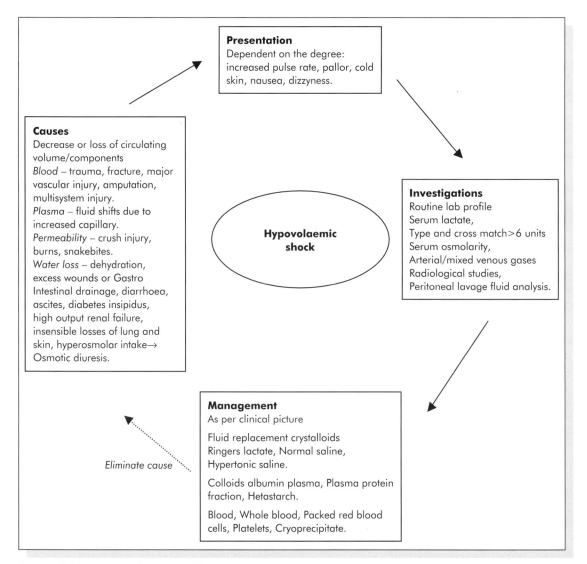

Figure 7.2 Management of hypovolaemic shock

Maureen O'Reilly

Shock can be classified according to four stages:

- stage I/early;
- stage II/moderate;
- stage III/major or progressive;
- stage IV/severe, profound, late, irreversible or uncompensated shock.

Specific management for the different types of shock are found in Figures 7.2–7.6 (pp. 110–114). The many and varied injury patterns mean that trauma patients may develop any of these types of shock.

HEAD AND SPINAL INJURY

Injuries to the head and spinal cord are categorized in two ways:

- whether the injury is primary and secondary;
- the site/s of injury/ies.

Primary injury patterns involve blunt or penetrating insult, as well as acceleration and or deceleration mechanisms and coup and or contrecoup patterns. Secondary injury occurs from hypoxia, hypercarbia, hypotension, intracranial hypertension. Spinal cord

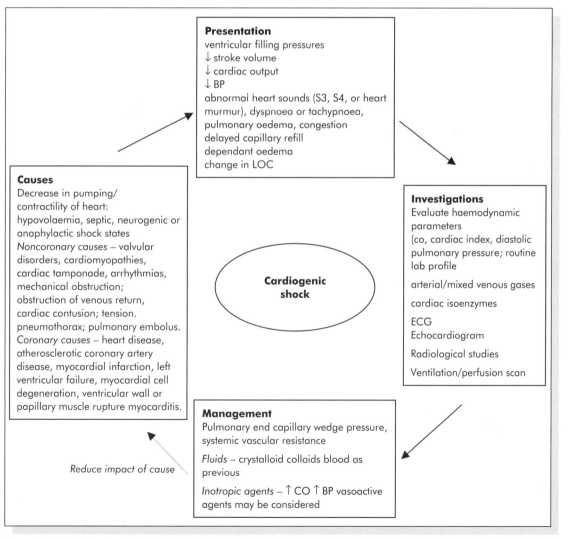

Presentation
ventricular filling pressures
↓ stroke volume
↓ cardiac output
↓ BP
abnormal heart sounds (S3, S4, or heart murmur), dyspnoea or tachypnoea, pulmonary oedema, congestion
delayed capillary refill
dependant oedema
change in LOC

Causes
Decrease in pumping/ contractility of heart:
hypovolaemia, septic, neurogenic or anaphylactic shock states
Noncoronary causes – valvular disorders, cardiomyopathies, cardiac tamponade, arrhythmias, mechanical obstruction; obstruction of venous return, cardiac contusion; tension. pneumothorax; pulmonary embolus.
Coronary causes – heart disease, atherosclerotic coronary artery disease, myocardial infarction, left ventricular failure, myocardial cell degeneration, ventricular wall or papillary muscle rupture myocarditis.

Cardiogenic shock

Investigations
Evaluate haemodynamic parameters
(co, cardiac index, diastolic pulmonary pressure; routine lab profile

arterial/mixed venous gases

cardiac isoenzymes

ECG
Echocardiogram

Radiological studies

Ventilation/perfusion scan

Reduce impact of cause

Management
Pulmonary end capillary wedge pressure, systemic vascular resistance

Fluids – crystalloid colloids blood as previous

Inotropic agents – ↑ CO ↑ BP vasoactive agents may be considered

Figure 7.3 Management of cardiogenic shock

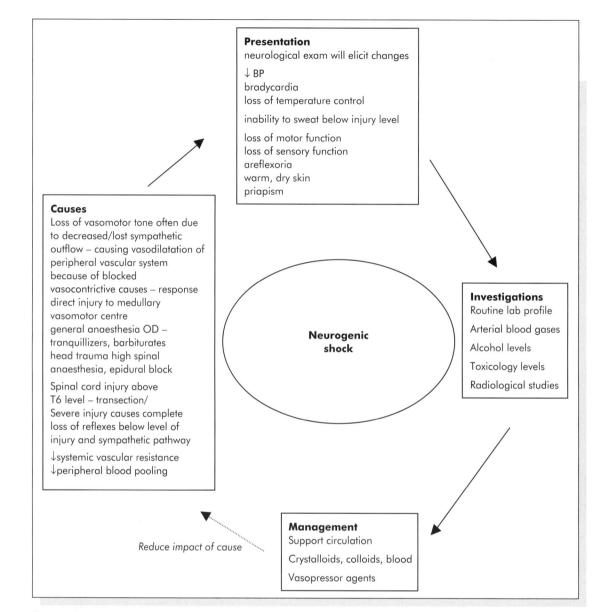

Presentation
neurological exam will elicit changes

↓ BP
bradycardia
loss of temperature control

inability to sweat below injury level

loss of motor function
loss of sensory function
areflexoria
warm, dry skin
priapism

Causes
Loss of vasomotor tone often due to decreased/lost sympathetic outflow – causing vasodilatation of peripheral vascular system because of blocked vasocontrictive causes – response direct injury to medullary vasomotor centre
general anaesthesia OD – tranquillizers, barbiturates head trauma high spinal anaesthesia, epidural block

Spinal cord injury above T6 level – transection/ Severe injury causes complete loss of reflexes below level of injury and sympathetic pathway

↓systemic vascular resistance
↓peripheral blood pooling

Neurogenic shock

Investigations
Routine lab profile

Arterial blood gases

Alcohol levels

Toxicology levels

Radiological studies

Reduce impact of cause

Management
Support circulation

Crystalloids, colloids, blood

Vasopressor agents

Figure 7.4 Management of neurogenic shock

injuries can also be caused by flexion, hyperextension, or vertical compression mechanisms.

The goal is to prevent further injury, compromise or deterioration. From the outset, it is important to be mindful of the physical, mental, emotional and social adjustments the injured individual must undergo for the remainder of their life. If the patient is aware of his injuries, it is possible that he and his family may start thinking and asking about these implications in the Emergency Department. Rapid, accurate and systematic neurological assessment will initially identify the *extent of the injuries*. History obtained from the patient, relatives and onlookers will assist in the *diagnosis of the injury*.

Maureen O'Reilly

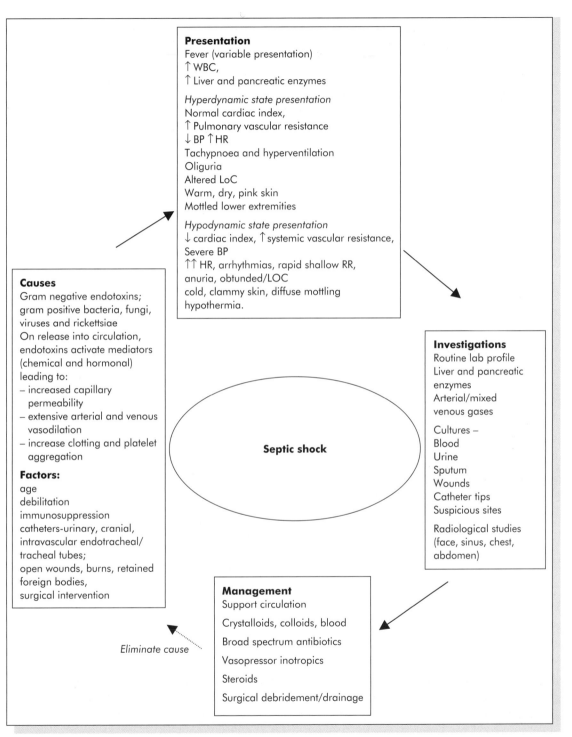

Presentation
Fever (variable presentation)
↑ WBC,
↑ Liver and pancreatic enzymes

Hyperdynamic state presentation
Normal cardiac index,
↑ Pulmonary vascular resistance
↓ BP ↑ HR
Tachypnoea and hyperventilation
Oliguria
Altered LoC
Warm, dry, pink skin
Mottled lower extremities

Hypodynamic state presentation
↓ cardiac index, ↑ systemic vascular resistance,
Severe BP
↑↑ HR, arrhythmias, rapid shallow RR,
anuria, obtunded/LOC
cold, clammy skin, diffuse mottling
hypothermia.

Causes
Gram negative endotoxins;
gram positive bacteria, fungi,
viruses and rickettsiae
On release into circulation,
endotoxins activate mediators
(chemical and hormonal)
leading to:
– increased capillary
  permeability
– extensive arterial and venous
  vasodilation
– increase clotting and platelet
  aggregation
Factors:
age
debilitation
immunosuppression
catheters-urinary, cranial,
intravascular endotracheal/
tracheal tubes;
open wounds, burns, retained
foreign bodies,
surgical intervention

Investigations
Routine lab profile
Liver and pancreatic
enzymes
Arterial/mixed
venous gases

Cultures –
Blood
Urine
Sputum
Wounds
Catheter tips
Suspicious sites

Radiological studies
(face, sinus, chest,
abdomen)

Septic shock

Management
Support circulation

Crystalloids, colloids, blood

Broad spectrum antibiotics

Vasopressor inotropics

Steroids

Surgical debridement/drainage

Eliminate cause

Figure 7.5 Management of septic shock

Major trauma management

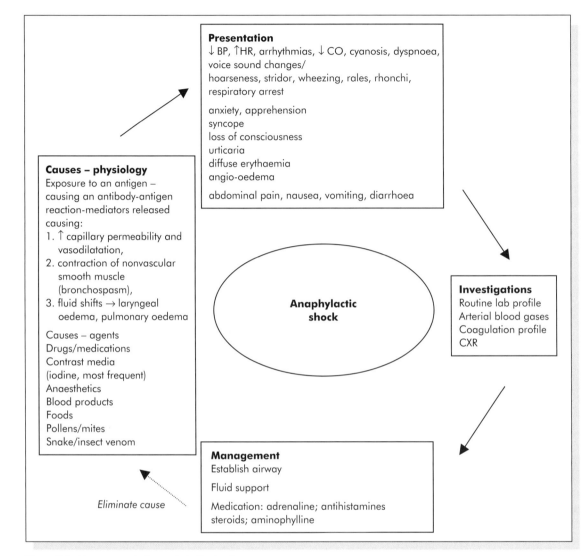

Presentation
↓ BP, ↑HR, arrhythmias, ↓ CO, cyanosis, dyspnoea, voice sound changes/ hoarseness, stridor, wheezing, rales, rhonchi, respiratory arrest

anxiety, apprehension
syncope
loss of consciousness
urticaria
diffuse erythaemia
angio-oedema

abdominal pain, nausea, vomiting, diarrhoea

Causes – physiology
Exposure to an antigen – causing an antibody-antigen reaction-mediators released causing:
1. ↑ capillary permeability and vasodilatation,
2. contraction of nonvascular smooth muscle (bronchospasm),
3. fluid shifts → laryngeal oedema, pulmonary oedema

Causes – agents
Drugs/medications
Contrast media
(iodine, most frequent)
Anaesthetics
Blood products
Foods
Pollens/mites
Snake/insect venom

Anaphylactic shock

Investigations
Routine lab profile
Arterial blood gases
Coagulation profile
CXR

Management
Establish airway

Fluid support

Medication: adrenaline; antihistamines steroids; aminophylline

Eliminate cause

Figure 7.6 Management of anaphylactic shock

HEAD INJURY ASSESSMENT

The assessment processes begins prior to arrival in the Emergency Department at the scene of injury. The prehospital care provider will obtain as much information as possible about

- patient position,
- interventions,
- behaviour/cognition/motor activity

both at the time of injury and through to transfer in the Emergency Department.

Level of consciousness – continual reassessment is required. Consciousness depends on arousal, a brainstem function and cognition of awareness, a cerebral hemisphere function.

Pupil assessment – small pinpoint penlight technique to each eye separately as a direct source to check direct/optic nerve response and indirect/consensual/occulomotor nerve response is done.

Drainages present assessment of the ear canal and nares for the presence of fluid or blood. These fluids can indicate communicating injuries and should be tested for the presence of cerebrospinal fluid. A halo of golden serous fluid will encircle a supply of blood on filter paper indicating the presence of cerebrospinal fluid.

Additional assessment

Length of amnesia

The more impairment of short-term memory/recent memory the more ominous the indication of injury.

Positioning

Abnormal flexion, abnormal extension or *flaccidity* indicate increased brain injury.

Muscle strength

The type and patterns of weakness, or the muscle groups that show patterns of weakness can elicit diagnostic clues.

Head injuries are classified into focal, brain injury, diffuse brain injury and skull fractures. Cerebral contusion and haematomas (epidural, subdural and intracerebral) are types of focal injury. Concussion and diffuse axonal injury are diffuse brain injury patterns. The symptoms, management and likely outcomes for these types of head injury are presented in Tables 7.1, 7.2a and 7.2b (pp. 116–118).

The incidence depends on

- the mechanism of injury,
- forces involved,
- injuring instrument,
- age of the patient.

Linear fractures are non-depressed; the force is distributed over a wide area. These are of no consequence unless the fracture is located near the temporal (middle meningeal artery), occipital/basilar/foramen magnum areas. These usually heal in 2–3 months.

Open/depressed fractures are complicated. The energy force is applied over a narrow area. The consequences include underlying tissue damage, bleeding and infection.

Basilar fractures occur at the base of the skull, result in direct communication to the cerebral hemisphere and cranial vault. There is a greater risk of brain abscess formation and cerebrospinal fluid leakage. The bones involved are: frontal, ethmoid, sphenoid, temporal or occipital bones.

Raised intracranial pressure is the complication of head trauma or spinal cord injuries that causes most concern. The intracranial cavity is composed of brain tissue (80%), blood (10%) and cerebrospinal fluid (10%). The Monro–Kellie hypothesis, or box theory, illustrates that any increase in one component must be accompanied by adjustments/decreases in one or both of the other components, or an overall increase in intracranial pressure will occur.

Intracranial pressure normally is 0–15 mmHg. Increased intracranial pressure has been identified as pressures greater than 15–20 mmHg. The clinical picture presents as early and late patterns of signs:

Early signs	Late signs
Headache	Cushing's Triad
Vomiting	Wide, pulse pressure/rising
↑ Systolic pressure	Decreasing heart rate
Papilloedema	
Abnormal respiratory pattern, depending on the site of the lesion	

Clinical management focuses on

- airway management,
- fluid management,
- control of the metabolic rate.

SPINAL CORD INJURY

Although there is an overall low incidence of spinal cord injury, there are significant social and financial impacts on the individual, family and community. Survival rates and morbidity levels have improved over the past few decades, however, the factors receiving most attention continue to be level of injury/lesion, extent of paralysis, age at time of injury/lesion, and survival of the first 3 months after the injury.

Primary injuries include deformation of the cord, rupture +/or occlusion of micro-vasculature, haemorrhage, decreased blood flow, loss of vascular autoregulation, oedema, necrosis.

Secondary injuries occur due to cell wall destruction, axonal swelling, vasoconstriction of spinal blood vessels, profound cord tissue hypoxia, haematoma formation and ultimate white matter necrosis.

Major trauma management

Table 7.1
Diffuse head injuries

Injury	Level of consciousness	Presentation	Diagnosis	Management and outcome
Concussion Mild	Temporary neuro dysfunction No LOC Momentarily dazed	Transient loss of: Consciousness Reflexes Respirations Amnesia	Neurological examination	Observation Discharge with carer
Severe	Temporary neuro dysfunction LOC Amnesia	Other symptoms: headache dizziness confusion irritability drowsiness visual disturbances	Neurological examination and X-ray	Admit for observation
Mild diffuse axonal injury	Coma lasting 6–24 h	Hypertension: SBP 140–160 Diencephalic involvement Transient posturing	CT scan	Medical management Mortality: 15% Good outcome: 80%
Moderate diffuse axonal injury	Coma lasting days to weeks	Hyperthermia: 35–40°C Hypothalamic dysfunction Subsides and re-occurs sporadically Posturing	CT scan	Medical management Mortality: 24%
Severe diffuse axonal injury	Coma begins at moment of impact Emergence by 3 months or increased vegetative state Signs of severe cerebral and brainstem dysfunction are present on admission or within 24 h	Hyperhidrosis Excessive sweating Occurs on face, less frequently on neck and thorax Sympathetically mediated Posturing	CT scan Small haemorrhagic lesions May be missed on early CT and resolve early Diffuse cerebral oedema Later: cerebral oedema and ventricular dilation	Medical management Mortality: 51%

Table 7.2a
Focal head injuries

Type of injury	LOC	Motor	Other	Treatment
Contusion (cortical bruising)	LOC Confusion		Deficit depends on location	Monitor for changes
Epidural/extradural haematoma (bleed between the dura and skull)	Initial LOC Lucid period Rapid deterioration	Contralateral hemiparesis	Headache Seizures Vomiting	Evacuation of haematoma
Acute subdural haematoma (bleed between the dura and arachnoid)	Confusion Drowsiness	Contralateral hemiparesis	Headache Agitation	Evacuation of haematoma Allow to reabsorb itself
Chronic subdural haematoma	Confusion Drowsiness	Contralateral hemiparesis (late)	Headache Seizure Papilloedema	Evacuation of haematoma Allow to reabsorb itself
Intracerebral haematoma	Decreased LOC progressing to coma	Contralateral hemiplegia	Headache Tentorial herniation	Allow to reabsorb

A common feature across different types of focal head injury is ipsilateral pupil dilation. Diagnosis is confirmed through CT scan.

The vertebral skeletal system is composed of the bone segments, ligaments and discs. The spinal cord is covered by the dura mater, arachnoid mater and pia mater. The subarachnoid space and central spinal canal contain cerebrospinal fluid. The cord grey matter is composed of nerve cell bodies, processes and fibres. The white matter contains the axons of the cells from the grey matter, axons of the dorsal column sensory cells, and descending tracts from the brain, brainstem or cerebellum. Myelination gives the white matter its appearance.

In addition to the neurological assessment already discussed; blood pressure, heart rate and rhythm, respiration rate and pattern, fluid intake, urine/vomit/faecal output monitoring and arterial blood gas trends need continual reassessment. Temperature evaluation will also need to be ongoing to detect and prevent the hypothermia due to peripheral vasodilation and loss of temperature-regulating ability.

The mechanism or patterns of injury include:

1 *Pure flexion* – results in sheared posterior ligaments, avulsion of spinous process frequently the vertebral body is wedged/dislocated anteriorly and there is spinal cord compression.

2 *Flexion and hyperflexion* – the more forceful impact is on the anterior vertebrae, multiple fragments are driven posteriorly causing dislocation of the vertebrae.

3 *Flexion with rotation* – usually has more fragment displacement of the vertebral body, with rupture of the posterior ligament system, the rotational component causes even greater cord compression.

4 *Hyperextension* – causes rupture of the anterior ligament causing fractured pedicles or body, causing additional dislocation and cord compression – also referred to by the lay population as hangman's fracture.

5 *Hyperextension with/followed by hyperflexion* – is frequently called whiplash.

6 *Hyperextension with rotation* – pedicle fractures, rupture of the anterior ligament system – and again rotational component causing even greater cord compression.

7 *Vertical compression* – loading injuries, more commonly occurring in blows, falls, tumours, osteomyelitis and Paget's Disease. Vertebral body compression, multiple fragments occur, increasing the spinal cord compression.

Table 7.2b
Focal head injuries

Causes	Clinical presentation	Management
Epidural/Extradural Haemorrhage (between the dura mater and the skull, usually the middle meningeal artery)		

Falls
Assaults
Motor vehicle crashes
	Depends on the source and
	  rapidity of the bleed
	Early sign: improved conscious level
	Later signs: rapid deterioration of level
	  of consciousness ipsilateral pupil
	  dilatation, contralateral hemiparesis,
	  headache, seizures, vomiting,
	  restlessness, diminished/slowing heart
	  rate rising systolic blood pressure,
	  variable respiratory pattern depending
	  on the site of injury
	60% present with clinical manifestations
	  within 6 or less hours
	Patient outcome is dependent on the
	  initial Glasgow Coma Score, the higher
	  the score the better the outcome
		CT scan head
		Treatment initially includes surgical
		  closure of the ruptured vessel/s

Subdural Haemorrhage (between the dura matter and arachnoid membranes)		

Falls
Assaults
Motor vehicle crashes
Shaking syndrome
  (child and elder abuse)
	Headache and confusion
	Decreasing level of consciousness
	  (as the reticular activation system
	  is affected)
		CT scan
		Evacuation of the haematoma for
		  lesions 3 mm or larger or clots of
		  10–400 ml
		Surgical intervention to control the
		  haemorrhage and resection of
		  the contused non-viable tissue
		Complications include increased
		  intracranial pressure, clot
		  reoccurrence, delayed
		  intracranial haemorrhage,
		  seizures
		The ultimate outcome is related to
		  the severity of the bleed and
		  early surgical intervention

Intracerebral Haematoma (a well-defined blood clot deep in the brain tissue or parenchyma)		

Traumatic causes
Shearing, causing diffuse
  axonal injury pattern,
  contusions, open/penetrating
  trauma
	Dependent on the size and location
	  of the haematoma
	The level of consciousness deteriorates
	  and progresses to coma
	Increased morality with co-existent
	  disseminated intravascular coagulation (DIC),
	  hypoxia, hypotension and alcohol abuse
		The goal is to allow reabsorption
		  to occur
		Frontal or temporal lobe
		  haematomas have a
		  90% morality

Vertebral injuries are classified in two ways

1 stable or unstable;
2 type of fracture.

Fractures are considered more stable if the surrounding support structures are limited in damage or if bony alignment is intact. Stable injuries rarely cause problems with spinal cord compromise, but early fusion/stabilization is generally undertaken to minimize the potential for neurological deficits.

Spinal cord injuries can occur primarily due to direct injury or secondarily due to concussion, contusion, haemodynamic changes, transection, damage to blood vessels that supply the cord and lastly biochemical changes. These are further defined as follows:

Concussion – temporary loss of function, can last 24–48 h; occurs in shaking syndromes; no permanent neurological changes occur.

Contusion – bruising of cord, bleeding into cord with oedema, potential necrosis. Permanent or extent of deficits are dependent on the severity of the contusion and necrosis.

Haemodynamic changes – the loss of the auto regulation mechanism causes decreased blood flow in the cord and results in cord ischaemic injury.

Transection – the cord is severed, is further defined as complete (rarely occurring) or incomplete. These are identified as physical (rare) or physiological (commonly seen) transections.

Anterior spinal and posterior spinal artery – injuries cause ischaemia and necrosis. This is sometimes referred to as "spinal cord stroke" by the lay population. Ischaemic changes can cause temporary deficits, whereas necrosis causes permanent changes.

Biochemical derangements can occur due to lactic acidosis, and the resultant effect of vasoconstriction and vasospasm furthering cord ischaemia.

Spinal cord injuries are further defined as follows:

Complete – where there is no preserved sensori-motor function below the level of injury.

Incomplete – where there is preservation of some sensori-motor fibres below the level of injury/lesion with varying degrees of function remaining.

Root injuries – are those that impair function of the motor/sensory system along a specific roots distribution path.

Spinal shock occurs immediately after spinal cord injury. The patient presents with flaccid paralysis; absent reflexes; loss of all pain, temperature, touch, proprioception and pressure below the level of injury/lesion; impaired/absent thermoregulation. Spinal shock can last from hours to weeks. Some patients may complain of severe pain in the "zone of heightened sensitivity" just above the level of injury. Other changes include: absent somatic/visceral sensations below the level of the lesion; bowel distension, absence of peristalsis, commonly seen in high cervical injuries – bradycardia, hypotension, venous pooling of the lower extremities. Spinal shock resolves as neurons regain excitability. The peri-anal reflexes return first.

Management of spinal cord injuries begins with *immobilization*. Temporary immobilization is based on injury type and spinal stability. Cervical methods include tongs (Gardner-Wells, Vinke, Crutchfield, Triple-Wells); skeletal traction in bed on bed/backboard; skeletal traction with roto-rest kinetic treatment bed, Stryker or Foster frames. Longer utilization methods include the foam collar; rigid collar; sternal-occipital-mandibular immobilizer; or halovest/brace. In the thoracic and lumbar area one sees skeletal-tibial pins (Halo-femoral traction) and progression to body casts/fibreglass jackets, canvas jacket, corset-like brace, Jewett brace, Knight–Taylor brace or more recently early spinal fusion of the injured level. Sacral or coccygeal spine injuries are treated with bed rest and girdle-like braces.

Pharmacological management includes:

Steroids – to reduce spinal cord oedema.

Osmotic diuretics – also used to reduce oedema often given with plasma expanders (e.g. Dextran) to support capillary cord flow.

Sodium bicarbonate – to maintain cerebrospinal fluid ph to decrease ischaemic acidosis.

Gastric antacids/histamine (H2) blockers – to prevent gastric ulcers.

Atropine – as needed for severe/symptomatic bradycardia.

Fluid management is cautious, hypotension is treated by stabilizing the cardiovascular system using vasopressors to attain/maintain a mean arterial pressure of 80 mmHg or higher. Respiratory management is crucial to outcomes. High flow humidified oxygen delivery is the minimum, continuous positive airway pressure (CPAP) and intubation/tracheostomy with mechanical ventilation using either negative or positive pressure ventilation is utilized. Long-term phrenic nerve pacing and diaphragmatic pacing may be instituted at some point.

Early surgical intervention is indicated for cord compression, evolving/extending deficits, compound vertebral fractures, penetrating spinal cord wounds or bone fragments are noted in the spinal canal.

CHEST TRAUMA

CARDIOTHORACIC TRAUMA

Chest injuries follow central nervous system injury as a leading cause of death in trauma. This can involve injuries to the heart, lung, lower airways, vascular structures and any component of the bony thorax. The mechanism can be a direct anatomical injury or alterations caused in physiological function. Assessment of the cardiothoracic patient includes physical assessment techniques of inspection, palpation, percussion and auscultation.

Rib fractures

Rib fractures are more frequently caused by blunt trauma mechanics. Clinically one sees decreased minute ventilation due to splinting from pain, ineffective ventilation causing atelectasis and hypoxia, and both enhancing secretion retention.

This injury pattern can be defined as

- fractures of one rib, simple;
- fractures of one rib, complicated (haemothorax or pneumothorax present);
- multiple rib fractures with stable chest wall (pulmonary contusions can be present);
- multiple rib fractures with instability of chest wall (pulmonary contusion, haemothorax and/or pneumothorax present);
- fractures of first rib associated with clavicle, fracture of second rib, fracture;
- scapula, lacerations of subclavian artery and/or vein and aortic rupture;
- fractures of left lower ribs (concurrent splenic injury a consideration);
- fractures of right lower ribs (concurrent liver injury a consideration);
- sternal fracture associated with pulmonary contusion and/or cardiac contusion.

Signs and symptoms can include chest wall pain that increases with deep breathing or coughing, localized tenderness on palpation, noted shallow respiratory effort, free movement at site, crepitus at site. Diagnosis is by chest and rib X-rays.

Treatment ranges from an intercostal nerve block, pain medication administration and incentive spirometry to intubation, mechanical ventilation and positive end expiratory pressure (PEEP) in the more severe cases. One no longer utilizes rib belts/binders or external skeletal traction as intervention modes. Healing generally takes 6–8 weeks.

Flail chest

Flail chest is an injury of two or more rib fractures; they can be adjacent or not, anterior, lateral or posterior. Some literature includes a sternal fracture in this category. The common denominator is loss of thorax/chest wall integrity. The fractured/flail segments no longer move in conjunction with changes in intrapleural pressure. The segment appears free-floating. Paradoxical movement is identified as an inward chest wall movement during inspiration and outward movement during expiration. This change causes alveolar tissue under the fracture segment to be compressed causing pulmonary physiologic shunting, mixing of venous and arterial blood and oxygen de-saturation.

Clinical findings occur as the bellows effect of the chest is lost and intrapleural pressure is less negative than normal. In addition to paradoxical chest wall movement, one sees increased respiratory rate and effort, and hypoxia, palpation of crepitus/fracture, pain on inspiration and palpation, decreased or absent breath sounds on injured side, dyspnoea, tachypnoea and respiratory failure can occur. External injury may be present – including abrasions, lacerations or bruising.

The treatment goal is to maintain PaO_2 at 11.5–13.5 kPa. Field management of the flail segment includes inclining the patient to the injured side. In the emergency/trauma setting, intubation and internal fixation via mechanical ventilation; controlled-CMV, assist-control (AC), or intermittent-control (IMU) with PEEP or CPAP is utilized. This modality is referred to as internal pneumatic stabilization. The decision for extent of interventions is dependent upon the size of the flail, amount of pulmonary dysfunction present, work of breathing, evidence of fatigue and the presence of concurrent thoracic injury.

Maureen O'Reilly

Pneumothorax

Pneumothorax is an injury where air is present in the pleural space due to rupture of alveoli/air sacs. Normal negative (intrapulmonary or intrapleura sub-atmospheric) pressure is lost and the lung on the affected side collapses. Depending on the mechanism of injury it can be unilateral or bilateral. The collapse leads to less area for ventilation and perfusion to occur, hypoxia results.

Clinical appearance is dependent on the extent of injury (partial, total collapse):

- asymptomatic,
- dyspnoea may be present,
- hyper-resonance on percussion on the affected sides,
- decrease or absence of breath sounds can occur,
- in extensive cases, subcutaneous emphysema can be present.

Diagnosis is confirmed by chest X-ray.

Treatment includes insertion of a chest tube. The 4th or 5th intercostal space, mid-axillary line is preferred in the adult patient. The 4th or 5th intercostal space or nipple line, anterior axillary line is the preferred site in children. This is connected to an underwater seal drainage system and the lung is monitored by chest X-ray for re-expansion.

Tension pneumothorax

Tension pneumothorax is a life-threatening condition and requires immediate intervention. Air enters the pleural space and is trapped without exit, in effect making a one-way valve system. Air continues to collect on each inspiration but cannot exit on expiration; compression of thoracic organs (trachea, lung, heart, mediastinum/great vessels). As the pressure increases, the compression may affect first one side of the chest cavity and progresses to both. The ultimate outcome is absence/failure to ventilate, absence of venous return, and decreasing to loss of cardiac output. The causes can be blunt or penetrating trauma, unresolved pneumothorax, bronchial tear, barotrauma, fractures ribs, tracheal injuries or pulmonary cyst.

The clinical signs and symptoms include:

- restlessness,
- extreme anxiety,
- hypoxia,
- severe air hunger,
- dyspnoea,
- tachypnoea,
- retraction,
- decreased or absent breath sounds on the affected side,
- tracheal deviation away from the affected side,
- hypertympany on percussion.

Other physiological changes may include decreasing cardiac output, hypotension, tachycardia, in the absence of hypovolaemia-distended neck veins, arterial blood gases indicate a rapid drop in PaO_2. Think *tension pneumothorax* in a patient with shock state and no other explainable causes of injury.

Treatment includes:

1 immediate needle decompression using at least a 14 gauge needle by inserting it *above* the 2nd intercostal space rib margin, mid-clavicular line (this avoids intercostal and internal mammary blood vessels);
2 insertion of one or more chest tubes that are attached to waterseal drainage;
3 definitive identification and treatment of the cause of tension pneumothorax.

Open pneumothorax

Open pneumothorax which has also been called "sucking chest wound", is due to penetrating trauma. The opening in the chest wall allows the equalization of intrathoracic and atmospheric pressure, again loss of negative pressure in the thorax occurs. It also allows air to move in and out the wound not allowing normal gas exchange to occur.

Clinical appearance includes a visible chest wall (anterior *or* posterior) defect persistent hole, restlessness, hypoxia, dyspnoea, tachypnoea, cyanosis, asymmetrical chest expansion, and gas bubbles/or audible abnormal gas movement may occur at the site of injury. Again this causes collapse of the same side lung.

Immediate treatment includes application of a sterile occlusive dressing, taped on 3 sides to allow a flutter/escape valve for air during expiration over the persistent hole/false airway. Treatment continues with the insertion of a chest tube on the *same side* of the injury but at *another site*. Corrective action includes surgical correction of defect. Constant observation for continued air collection in the pleural space, barotrauma and tension pneumothorax is indicated.

Haemothorax

Haemothorax is a collection of blood in the pleural space. Injury to chest wall vessels, internal mammary arteries, or intercostal arteries and their accompanying veins. Penetrating wounds can cause injury to major pulmonary vessels, any of the mediastinal structures or diaphragm. Blunt or iatrogenic injury can also occur. Most often major bleeding is not due to lung parenchymal injury. A massive haemothorax is identified as a collection of 1.5–4.0 l of blood in the pleural space. Left sided haemothorax is frequently caused by rib fracture, injuries to: pulmonary parenchymal, aortic isthmus, spleen, heart, intercostal artery, supra-aortic vessel, major pulmonary vessel or the diaphragm (in descending order of frequency). Right-sided haemothorax (also in descending order of frequency) is caused by rib fracture, injury to: pulmonary parenchyma, liver, intercostal/internal mammary artery, supra-aortic vessel, pulmonary vessel, aortic isthmus, heart, diaphragm.

Clinical presentation is of dyspnoea, shortness of breath, decreased or absent breath sounds on the side of haemothorax, dullness on percussion, tracheal deviation *away* from affected side, hypoxia, shock symptoms, flat neck veins and mediastinal shift. Diagnostic studies include chest X-ray.

Treatment includes cardiovascular support, insertion of a *large* bore chest tube (30–40 fv) into the 4th or 5th intercostal space, mid-axillary line (adults) to drain blood and air, monitoring drainage amount and replacement of blood loss. Timely surgical intervention is indicated. Autologous blood transfusion is possible via auto transfusion devices. The methods and equipment utilized need to be reviewed by staff to maintain skill and current knowledge.

Pulmonary contusion

Pulmonary contusion is often a compression/decompression injury that results in bruising of lung tissue. This can be mild to severe in classification. It is a two prong process with haemorrhagic and oedematous effects (interstitial and alveolar).

The dynamics can be graphed as follows:

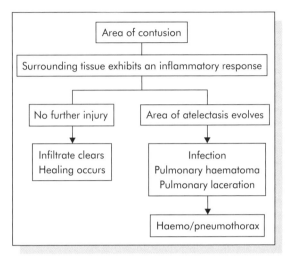

It is commonly caused by deceleration, blunt trauma or a high-velocity missile. Clinical signs and symptoms include: haemoptysis, fever, tachycardia, hypoxia, hypercarbia, wheezing, rales, tachypnoea, decrease in pulmonary compliance and increase in airway pressure. Chest X-ray will demonstrate a non-segmental whiteout.

Treatment is aimed at decreasing the pulmonary shunt – this is accomplished by oxygen administration, using the lowest FiO_2 necessary and augmenting functional residual capacity with PEEP. Lung compliance can be increased with the use of diuretics. Fluid restriction can be instituted in the absence of shock.

Cardiac contusion

Cardiac contusion is a bruising of heart tissue; the blunt injury can cause small oedematous areas of contusion to larger collections of blood/haemorrhage. The capillary haemorrhage causes separation and disruption of myocardial fibres. The overall effect is of decreased cardiac output and decreased inotropic effect.

The clinical presentation consists of precordial pain, not relieved with nitrates, external signs of trauma (contusion, lacerations), frequently tachycardia is present. Arrhythmias will also occur – multiple premature ventricular contractions (PVCs), ventricular tachycardia (VT), atrial fibrillation, or conduction defects/blocks. Other ECG abnormalities may be present indicating ischaemia. Serial cardiac enzymes and isoenzymes should be monitored. Complications include: cardiac tamponade, cardiogenic shock, myocardial rupture, fibrosis with/without ventricular aneurysm development, valvular injuries, or constrictive pericarditis.

Treatment is the same as a patient having a myocardial infarction-monitoring must continue for 48–72 h for arrhythmias. Additional studies may be done to evaluate ventricular wall movement and calculate ventricular ejection fractions.

Cardiac tamponade

Cardiac tamponade is life threatening and requires immediate treatment. This is an accumulation of blood in the non-distensible/tough pericardial sac. Normally 25 ml of fluid is present as a protective cushion for cardiac tissue. An injury introducing blood (or air), even in amounts as small as 50–100 ml, will produce an increase in intra-pericardial pressure.

The clinical presentation is based upon the rate of collection as well as total accumulation of fluid. Clinical presentation is known as Becks triad-systemic hypotension, muffled heart sounds and elevated venous pressure (distended neck veins). Pulsus paradoxus calculated at over 10–15 mmHg during inspiration is clinically significant. One can also see elevated CVP, narrowed pulse pressure, rapidly declining cardiac output. ECG changes can be noted in precordial leads – low voltage complexes will be noted. Air hunger and respiratory distress will be evident.

Diagnosis and treatment are accomplished by pericardio-centesis. Fluid is aspirated by 14–16 or 18 gauge angiocath/catheter-over-the-needle from the pericardial sac – the catheter is left in place and secured for necessary re-aspiration/return of symptoms. It is important to remember pericardial fluid does not clot as it is defibrinated by cardiac motion within the pericardium. The cause of the tamponade needs to be identified and corrected urgently. An emergent thoracotomy may be indicated.

Aortic/great vessel rupture/transection

Aortic/great vessel rupture/transection is a lethal injury. Over 90% die at the scene; usually a complete transection. Less than 80% survive past 6 h, these are incomplete transections or partial tears. Tears frequently occur at sites of anatomical fixation:

1 ligamentum arteriosum, distal to the origination of the left subclavian artery;
2 root of the aorta just above the aortic valve;
3 aortic hiatus at diaphragm;
4 innominate artery.

This injury is more often caused by blunt (acceleration/deceleration) and penetrating trauma.

Clinical presentation includes

- restlessness;
- dyspnoea;
- hoarseness from haematoma (producing pressure on laryngeal area);
- dysphagia from haematoma (producing pressure on the oesophageal area);
- stridor;
- pain that is retrosternal or interscapular in location;
- upper extremity hypertension;
- blood pressure and pulse differences in the upper extremities – including a palpable difference in pulse volume and amplitude in the upper and lower extremities.

Other physiological changes that may present include: decreased or absent femoral pulses, tachycardia, hypotension unexplained by other injuries, pallor, precordial or intra-scapular systolic murmur and lower extremity sensory and/or neuromuscular deficits.

Diagnosis is made on suspicion/mechanisms of injury, clinical findings, and chest X-ray abnormalities. On chest X-ray, one frequently sees a widened mediastinum, obliteration of the aortic knob, tracheal and oesophageal deviation to the right and pleural capping. Positioning of the patient in a supine or semi-erect position for the X-ray distorts the mediastinum, making it appear wider. Definitive diagnosis is usually confirmed by arteriogram of the aorta (aortography) – although chest CT scan and MRI may also be undertaken. Treatment in the Emergency Department includes: emergent surgical intervention, cardiopulmonary bypass or a shunt-bypass technique are used to permit resection and grafting.

ABDOMINAL AND GENITOURINARY TRAUMA

Abdominal and genitourinary (GU) trauma frequently are the most difficult to identify and are a common occurrence in trauma patients. Abdominal tenderness, haemodynamic instability, occurrence of lumbar spine injury, or pelvic fracture require additional investigation; as does the presence of free air on X-ray studies in the retro-peritoneal or intra-peritoneal areas.

The peritoneal cavity houses the stomach, small intestine, liver, gall bladder, spleen, transverse colon, sigmoid colon, upper third of rectum and reproductive female organs. The retro-peritoneal cavity contains part of the duodenum, ascending colon, descending colon, kidneys, pancreas and major vessels. The four quadrant division is most commonly used in the assessment process.

Inspection of the abdomen is sequenced: inspection, auscultation, percussion and palpation.

Diagnostic studies used in abdominal trauma include contrast studies, chest and abdominal X-rays, bedside and radiological ultrasound, CAT scan, MRI and arteriography. Haemoglobin, haematocrit, leukocyte counts, serum amylase and lipase levels are essential. Other tests sources include diagnostic peritoneal lavage, laporotomy and endoscopy procedures.

Oesophageal injury

Oesophageal injury can result from penetrating trauma, blunt trauma or caustic ingestion.

Signs and symptoms vary by site of rupture and amount of contamination by digestive juices and bacterial contamination. They include passive resistance to neck movement, dyspnoea, hoarseness, bleeding orally, cough, stridor, pain at the site of rupture/laceration, which may radiate to the neck, chest, shoulders or abdomen.

Gastric intubation with a Levine or Salem-sump tube is done to drain stomach contents, decompress the stomach and prevent aspiration. Lateral cervical spine films may show retro-oesophageal air. Surgical reconstruction of the oesophagus is the main stay of treatment.

Diaphragmatic injury

Diaphragmatic injury, especially the left hemidiaphragm, can occur due to blunt trauma. Diagnosis is often delayed or found during radiological studies for other abdominal or chest injuries. Bowel sounds may be heard in the chest; or on X-ray the presence of abdominal organs or the nasogastric tube in the chest may be seen. Changes in the shape of the right hemidiaphragm may indicate liver encroachment through the tear.

Treatment – intra-operative repair is indicated. Careful patient handling is essential to reduce increase in intra-abdominal pressure and prevent a small laceration from enlarging.

Liver trauma

Liver trauma is common due to the size and location of this organ. Injury occurs from blunt and penetrating mechanisms. Clinical findings can include pain/tenderness over the right lower six ribs, or right upper quadrant, dullness on percussion may be elicited. One can sometimes see an increasing abdominal girth on measurement. Symptom onset can be as late as 72 h post-injury.

Splenic trauma

Splenic trauma is common due to its size and location in the upper quadrant – again blunt trauma, deceleration patterns and penetrating trauma are the culprit. Clinical findings include – left upper quadrant pain, Kehr's sign, Ballance's sign, local tenderness, "spasm". The extent of haemodynamic instability varies with the amount of injury, time of insult to injury and the speed of blood loss. Clinical presentation can be of hypovolaemia and peritonitis.

Pancreatic injury

Pancreatic injury is less common and more often occurs due to penetrating trauma. The injury can be occult, especially in multi organ injuries. Symptom onset may be as late as 24 h post-injury. Clinical presentation includes abdominal tenderness over the pancreatic area, epigastric pain, guarding and Grey-Turner's sign. An index of suspicion is crucial for the appropriate diagnostic evaluation. Monitor for ileus development, elevation of serum amylase and lipase levels, hypovolaemia, and sepsis. Diagnostic peritoneal lavage is not helpful in the identification of pancreatic injury due to the retro-peritoneal bleed potential, and amylase may be in the fluid due to other organ injuries.

Stomach, duodenal, jejunum and ileum injuries

Stomach, duodenal, jejunum and ileum injuries are more frequently due to penetrating than blunt trauma. The injury patterns include perforation, rupture, transection or haematoma formation. Duodenal injuries often occur in conjunction with pancreatic, bile duct or vena cava trauma. Jejunum and ileum injuries occur more frequently injured proximally in the first, distally in the latter as they are fixation points anatomically. Since symptom onset can be delayed, an index of suspicion is important.

Clinical presentation can include nausea, vomiting, fever, jaundice, signs of high intestinal obstruction, pain in the epigastric or right lower quadrant regions, and testicular pain. Diagnostic testing include X-rays (90% – negative/non-specific findings) and CAT scans.

Large bowel, colon, rectal trauma

Large bowel, colon, rectal trauma are the most fatal of abdominal trauma, even though they account for only 5% of all abdominal traumas. Ninety-six per cent of these traumas are penetrating, increasing the risk of faecal contamination. Blunt trauma occurs in deceleration injury patterns. Consider delayed rupture as a potential problem even in contusion situations. An adequate history would include the events history, wounding agent, proximity to the implement/weapon-food and beverage consumption, and current tetanus immunization also play a role in outcomes.

Clinical signs and symptoms include – pain and tenderness on abdominal and rectal examination, evolving signs of peritonitis. Diagnosis may include diagnostic peritoneal lavage – chest and abdominal films, radiological studies with dye contrast, and CT scans are sometimes undertaken. An early laporotomy is indicated if the patient is showing signs of intra-abdominal bleeding.

Close monitoring for wound infection, development of haemorrhagic/septic shock and identification of associated injuries is crucial in the trauma resuscitation period.

Vascular injuries

Vascular injuries in the abdominal compartment do occur. They can present due to shearing, tearing or compression mechanisms as contusions, lacerations, transections or avulsion injuries. Avulsion injuries usually occur at sites of attachment – especially renal pedical, or the root of mesentery vessels.

These patients present in a shock state or may mimic visceral rupture and haemorrhage. In the latter case, complaints of back or abdominal pain are elicited, assessment may reveal hypoactive bowel sounds, or abdominal distension, haematuria or palpable tender mass. Delays usually occur in the development of flank discoloration or Grey-Turner's sign.

Overall, treatment is directed at control of bleeding, then and concurrent blood and fluid replacement. Two common sites of injury include the interior vena cava (at juxtahepatic, suprarenal, peri-renal and infra-renal sites) portal vein and the aorta. Diagnosis is attempted radiologically in the stable patient; Doppler flow studies may be added to the picture. Surgical repair is dependent upon venous or arterial source; closure, anastomosis, shunts or graphs may be indicated. On occasion nephrectomy may be indicated.

Genitourinary injuries

Genitourinary injuries include any injury to the kidney, collecting system or reproductive organs. It is more commonly present in association with other injuries; these include rib fractures, other abdominal injuries. The causes include blunt, penetrating and iatrogenic injuries. Throughout the literature in patients with congenitally abnormal kidneys, adhesions/strictures of renal system, history of kidney stones – chronic GU infection, renal failure, renal artery stenosis, or glomerulopathies, the incidence of renal injury is greater.

Overall inspection will assist in identifying potential GU injuries. Examination for Grey-Turner's sign, blood at the urinary meatus, an oedematous and/or contused scrotum or labia may be helpful. Female patients need evaluation for tampons, diaphragms or intrauterine devices to prevent septic complications. Haematuria, taught as the key sign or hallmark of GU trauma, is not always evident. Diagnosis is made based upon kidney–ureter–bladder (KUB) flat plate films, intravenous pyelogram (IVP), cystogram or urethrogram, nuclear imaging, ultrasound, tomography, renal angiography, and/or CAT scan results. If blood is noted at the urinary meatus-a urinary catheter should not be placed and a urethrogram must be performed.

Common injuries to the kidneys include contusion or rupture.

Ureteral injuries

Ureteral injuries are most often due to penetrating trauma. The mechanism of injury should heighten the index of suspicion; the patient may describe flank pain and present with haematuria. A laceration or contusion may appear on IVP studies. Treatment will include immediate surgical repair, and/or urinary diversion through the utilization of nephrostomy tubes or a ureterostomy. Ongoing evaluation of ureter patency, appropriate urine output, and collection of intra-urine is indicated. The latter is identified by fluid seepage through the sutures, abdominal girth enlargement or declining urine output.

Bladder injuries

Bladder injuries can occur due to blunt or penetrating trauma. The risk of injury is greater in a distended or full state – as tension increases over the dome (top) and weakest component of the bladder.

Clinical presentation can include the inability to void, haematuria, signs and symptoms of peritonitis. A rupture is almost always present in an acceleration–deceleration injury or fractured pelvis. Diagnosis is best accomplished through a urethrocystogram.

Minor wounds can be managed conservatively via decompression of the bladder (Urinary or supra-pubic catheters are effective), or intra-operative closure may be indicated in larger wounds.

Urethral injuries

Urethral injuries can occur from blunt and penetrating sources. This injury is often concurrent with pelvic fractures, or other GU injuries. The male is more susceptible and more commonly injured due to anatomical structures. No attempts should be made to insert a urinary catheter when an assessment indicates a suspected urethral injury.

Clinical signs include blood at the urinary meatus, a patient who is unable to void, or a bladder that is displaced and higher in the abdomen on palpation. On exam of the prostate it may appear "floaty" or

"absent", sometimes a "boggy" haematoma can be palpated.

Treatment includes diagnosis via an immediate urethrogram, then an insertion of a supra-pubic catheter/supra-pubic cystostomy. Males are at risk for genital injury to the testicles and penis from blunt, penetrating or de-gloving injuries. They can range from a fractured pelvis (rupture of the tumca albuginea), lacerations, amputation, crush, avulsions, strangulation, burns and rupture. Treatment may be surgical or conservative; with the goal to return the patient to full urinary and sexual function. Females are at greater risk to reproductive organs in penetrating injury. Assessment findings are usually of a peritonitis nature – especially in the non-pregnant state. Females are at risk for the same external genitalia injuries. The mechanisms for both include assault, aggressive sexual activity, industrial/agricultural accidents and the application or introduction of foreign bodies. A speculum exam should be performed in all females with pelvic injuries. Diagnostics include ultrasound, and CAT scans. Often an emergency laporotomy is performed in the unstable patient.

All abdominal, renal, GU and reproductive injuries are at risk for haemorrhage and infection/sepsis/intra-abdominal abscess formation. Other complications include adult respiratory distress syndrome (ARDS), pancreatitis, evisceration, thrombus formation, development of an ileus, and disruption of wound healing.

MUSCULOSKELETAL TRAUMA

Although extremity and skeletal injury may present as the most obvious trauma on a patient's arrival in the Emergency Department, it is not routinely addressed in the primary survey.

Musculoskeletal trauma is assessed in the secondary survey. As with all other sources of trauma, one can review common causes or mechanisms of injury and note falls, industrial/agricultural accidents, sports related injuries, assaults, or motor vehicle crashes. The issue can be further investigated by the concept of direct and indirect forces. Direct trauma results when forces of energy are absorbed at the impact site. This can be further delineated into

Maureen O'Reilly

tapping fractures, crush fractures and penetrating or impalement injuries. Indirect trauma is described when an impact causes damages distant from the point of impact.

Additional injury forces include muscle contraction, fatigue and pathological processes (rickets, Paget's disease and metastatic disease).

The injury patterns typically presenting in musculoskeletal areas include fractures, dislocations, subluxations, strains, sprains and amputations.

The assessment process includes:

inspection,
palpation,
percussion, and
auscultation.

Inspection for skin colour, (pale-arterial interruption, dusky-venous alteration), bruising/bleeding; evidence of muscle spasms (continuous muscle contractions); swelling (indicating soft tissue injury venous or lymphatic disruption); position of the extremity (evidence of anatomical alignment or deformity); open or closed fracture present; the presence of skin defects (abrasions, lacerations or avulsions) or impaled objects.

Palpation allows assessment of skin temperature, capillary refill times, the presence-quality-equality of pulses, specific point elicited tenderness, muscle spasm, active and passive range of motion – to identify limitations or abnormalities, noting the feel/presence of crepitus, and peripheral nerve assessment for motor strength and sensory intactness.

Percussion is utilized in the assessment of deep tendon reflexes.

Auscultation will elicit vital signs, and the presence of a bruit over vessels in an injured area.

In view of the complex assortment of orthopaedic injuries that present in the Emergency Department, it is helpful to review mechanisms of injury. The injuries may be caused by tapping/direct deceleration force over a small area, crush pattern, penetrating injury (projectiles or impalement), or indirect trauma (impact elsewhere causes the problem). The injury can be initiated by fall, sport/contact mechanism, assaults or vehicular crashes. Identification of different types of injury is presented in Table 7.3 (pp. 128–131).

Complications of orthopaedic injuries begins early in the injury process. Constant reassessment for vascular or neurological compromise is imperative. Evaluation of the "six P's" is routinely undertaken:

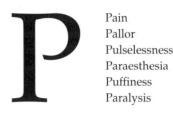

P
Pain
Pallor
Pulselessness
Paraesthesia
Puffiness
Paralysis

Compartment syndrome – pressures increase between sheaths/sheets of fascia from internal or external sources. Normal compartmental pressure is less than 20 mmHg. It can be measured continuously or by single measurement techniques. Early symptoms include throbbing pressure, taut muscle stretch, pain out of proportion to the injury on passive range of motion or flexion. Late signs – diminished limb mobility, paralysis and loss of pulse. Fasciotomy would be the normal course of treatment. If untreated, muscle death, loss of the limb, myoglobinuria and renal complications may occur.

Initial care and prevention with early stabilization of bone fragments, supplemental oxygen administration and fluid replacement is important. Monitoring early signs of the decreasing PaO_2 and change in mental state is key, as is monitoring for tachycardia; hypotension; increasing cardiac output and increasing pulmonary resistance. Chest pain or shortness of breath may be present. Chest X-ray will show bilateral fluffy infiltrates in the late stages.

Management of this syndrome is similar to ARDS and requires intubation, mechanical ventilation, application of PEEP, positioning of patient and support of the cardiovascular system. Renal changes can include – diguria, anuria, lipuria and haematuria. Skin assessment for flat red, appearing in waves of petechiae on trunk, axilla, chest, conjunctiva and mucous membranes is classical in this syndrome.

FACIAL, ENT, DENTAL TRAUMA

Facial trauma is known for increased incidence in trauma events. Both the anatomical structures and unprotected position of the face lead to this dilemma. The upper third of the facial structure contains the frontal sinus, frontal bone, glabella and supraorbital

Major trauma management

Table 7.3
Types of injury

	Signs/symptoms	Treatment	Diagnosis	Specific pattern
Location				
1. Musculotendinous strain – overstretching or weakening of muscle where attachment to tendon occurs	*Mild* – local pain point tenderness *Moderate* – above plus: swelling discolouration inability to use joint for long periods of time *Severe* – above plus: snapping sound at time of injury severely restricted range of motion *Rarely* – neurovascular changes	"RICE" Rest Immobilization – no weight bearing for at least 42 h/crutches Cold applications Compression – ace, air cast device Elevation	Negative X-rays	Achilles tendon – start and stop activities/sports Deformity of calf develops Simmonds test (ankle flexion with compression of calf muscle occurs with intact tendon) done, compression dressing, elevation onto heels, or surgery used
2. Ligamentous sprain – tearing of ligamentous fibres – actions exceeds normal range of motion	*First degree* – minor tear of ligament fibre–mild tenderness, bruising, slight decrease in range of motion *Second degree* – partial tear of ligament–above symptoms ⊕ point tenderness and swelling *Third degree* – complete tear of ligament – above symptoms ⊕ pain, loss of function, abnormal motion, possible deformity Neurovascular changes evident in an unstable joint	"RICE" Rest Immobilization – no weight bearing/ crutches/splinting device Cold applications Compression – ace, air cast device Elevation Aspiration of haemarthrosis if indicated Arthroscopy repair Physical therapy	Routine X-rays – negative Stress/weighted views – may show third degree sprain Arthrography Arthroscopy MRI CAT scan	Knee-drawer sign: instability with range of motion
3. Joint injuries contusion – inflammatory response subluxation – incomplete dislocation	Oedema, exudate, decreased range of motion Some articular contact in place, altered range of motion	Splint in position found No relocation/reduction of joint prior to hospital evaluation unless neurovascular	Routine X-rays – positive prior to reduction/relocation CAT scan	Sterno-clavicular pain/inability to abduct anterior dislocation – deformity Posterior dislocation – depression, vascular changes

Maureen O'Reilly

	Signs/symptoms	Treatment	Diagnosis	Specific pattern
dislocation – separation of two articular joint surfaces	Damage to joint capsule and torn ligament most often present Severe pain, joint deformity Swelling, point tenderness Significant decrease/change in range of motion	compromise present Rapid transport, rapid access to reduction/relocation Sling/swath, splinting devices, AC strap, surgical or closed reductions		Acromo-clavicular (AC) inability to raise arm or place across chest Shoulder – anterior – over 90% of pattern, arm abducted and externally rotated Posterior – more rare – arm abducted and internally rotated Look for flattened deltoid, lowered axilla area, prominence of acromnion process Elbow – anterior or posterior presentations, later most common – "locked elbow" evaluate for Volkman's ischaemic contracture Hip – inability to move shortened leg Anterior – external rotation, palpable femoral head Posterior – knee and hip flexion, sciatic nerve injury, **femoral artery compromise Knee – posterior, lateral, medial or hyperextension presentations – higher incidence of vascular and nerve damage Patellar – lateral deformity, knee held in flexion position Ankle – commonly associated with fracture Foot – tarsal and metatarsals can be affected – rare occurrences
Type of injury Fractures Classified by: a) **Cause** – pathological (diseased bone), stress/fatigue (unaccustomed or repeated activity), traumatic	Pain Point tenderness Deformity Swelling Bruising	Control bleeding Replace fluid loss: potential loss: Humerus – 500–1500 ml Elbow – 250–750 ml Radius/ulna – 250–500 ml	Plain X-rays AP, lateral views include joint above and below Children-comparison views Arteriogram/ angiogram CAT scan	Clavicle – assess for crepitus and head tilt towards the injured site Scapula – pain increases with abduction, bruising Shoulder – unable to move arm, arm held in adduction, gross swelling and discolouration Humerus-midshaft – shortening, abnormal mobility, crepitus, bruising

Major trauma management

Table 7.3 (continued)

Signs/symptoms	Diagnosis	Treatment	Specific pattern
b) **Closed or open** wound involving fracture site c) **Extent of fracture** complete – break extends through entire bone incomplete – partial break displaced – bone fragments separate from fracture line comminuted – three or more bone fragments at fracture line impacted – fracture line has been compressed or telescoped into itself overriding – complete fracture with ends of fracture overriding each other d) **Type of fracture** Longitudinal – same direction as long bone axis Transverse – 90° angle across bone shaft Oblique – 45° angle across bone shaft Spiral – similar to oblique, longer in length Compression – crush type, severe force, applied to head or heels Avulsion – bone breaks off at muscle insertion site Depressed – fracture area lower than surrounding bone	Bone scan Arthrogram	Pelvis – 750–6000 ml Femur – 500–3000 ml Tibia – 250–2000 ml Ankle – 250–1000 ml Immobilize as found if no vascular compromise present Stabilize fractures- closed reduction with splint, bandage or cast Open reduction internal fixation plates, screws, rods, etc. External fixator devices as appropriate	*Humerus-supracondylar* – unable to move elbow, deformity, fat pad sign may be present *Elbow* – pain on pronation and supination, joint effusion *Radius/ulna* – shaft distal forearm – *Colle's type* – dinner fork deformity (dorsal angulation) bruising *Distal forearm-Smith's type* – garden spade deformity (volvar angulation), lower end of radius protrudes *Scaphoid/navicular* – point tenderness in anatomic snuffbox – need navicular views or bone scan for best diagnosis *Hand-metacarpal fractures* – Point tenderness and swelling *Finger/phalangeal fractures* – subungal haematoma mallet finger – unable to extend finger *Pelvic fractures* – crepitus, tenderness at symphysis pubis/anterior spine/iliac crests sacrum/coccyx, inability to bear weight, unexplained shock, bruising (groin, flank, suprapubic/pelvic-perineal areas, bleeding from urethra/rectum/vagina, haematuria *Acetabulum fracture* – tenderness with movement, unable to bear weight *Hip fractures* External rotation and swelling, inability to bear weight *Femoral shaft fracture* – inability to bear weight, limb is shorter *Patella fractures* – look for haemarthrosis, crepitus, deformity *Tibia/fibula fracture* – inability to bear weight

Signs/symptoms	Treatment	Diagnosis	Specific pattern
			Ankle fractures – presentations: inversion-lateral malleolus Aversion-medial malleolus Impaction Posterior dislocation Overall, unable to bear weight Foot fractures – unable to bear weight – inversion tears base of metatarsal (5th, most common) Calcaneous/os calcis fracture – unable to bear weight, back pain if jumping/fall pattern Toe/metatarsal fracture – unable to bear weight
Amputated limb	Thorough cleansing Wrap amputated part in moist, sterile dressing place part in sterile plastic bag container Place wrapped part in insulated cooler with crushed ice Do not freeze part Do not place on dry ice Non-cooled ischaemia – extremity used to 6–8 h digit – 10–12 h With cooled ischaemia over 12 h, less than 24 h for reattachment Operating room debridement, stabilization of bone, reattachment	Assessment of affected limb and separated part crucial! Plain radiographs Doppler flow studies Assess for red line sign-capillary bleeding Reattachment may be contraindicated in severely crushed mangled injury, multilevel amputations previous serious injury, concurrent serious injury or atherosclerotic states	Each situation must be evaluated on an individual basis Photographic documentation if available Goal: functional use, not just cosmetics

ridge. The middle third/midface contains the orbit, maxillary sinuses, nose, vomer, zygoma, maxilla, palate, maxillary teeth and alveolar process. The lower third contains the mandible and mandibular teeth. Assessment includes inspection and palpation primarily.

Palpation for irregularities and deformities begins across the forehead, along supraorbital ridge, continues to the infraorbital ridge and zygong, comparing for depression of the zygomatic arch, and manoeuvring the maxilla to identify free motion.

Direct visualization for gross dental occlusion and alignment completes the process. The injury pattern can be caused by blunt or penetrating trauma as well as exposures to toxins (especially acids or alkalis). The more common injuries occur in the midface/ middle third area. These include the orbits, nose, zygoma, maxilla, and midface/La Forte Fractures. The mandible is also frequently injured.

BURN/THERMAL TRAUMA

Thermal trauma can be caused by sources:

heat – direct or indirect contact of the skin with a heat source of sufficient magnitude to coagulate the skin's protein component, causing coagulation necrosis and diminished or absent blood flow.

electrical – coagulation necrosis occurs from entry to exit sites and anywhere in between.

cold – this can be a localized tissue destruction/ frostbite or a core temperature change/ hypothermia.

Overall burns are the third most common injury seeking care in the Emergency Department. This does not account for the untabulated numbers of smaller burns not treated. Those at risk: extremes of ages, lower socio-economic status residents, and those in high risk occupations (in contact with liquid metal, tar, chemicals or intense heat).

The integumentary system (skin) is the largest organ in the body – provides protection against infection, prevents fluid loss, controls body temperature, secretes oils, excretes 30–50 ml/h water vapour in adults, produces vitamin D, determines an individual's cosmetic and cultural identity, is an organ of sensation and plays a role in the regeneration of new skin.

THERMAL BURNS

A cycle of injury quickly establishes with increased vascular permeability, fluid shifts and haemolysis:

1 *Increased vascular permeability* – occurs due to direct *heat-induced* endothelial cell injury; *mediator-induced* endothelial cell injury such as the potent vasodilators prostaglandin, histamine, bradykinin and oxygen radical arrive on the scene.

   Impaired vascular permeability occurs, there is loss of the osmotic pressure gradient, osmotic pressures climb to 200–300 mmHg, causing rapid water and protein shifts.

2 Fluid shifts occur intravascular to interstitial for the first 24–36 h – it is most apparent within 8 h. The capillary integrity starts to restore within that 24–36 h.

3 *Haemolysis* of the red blood cell causes an increase in free plasma haemoglobin, haemoglobinuria; with the shorter red blood cell life span, there is a concurrent decrease in haematocrit. The burn injury causes a decreased red blood cell manufacture which remains in effect until the burn wound closes. There is clinically concurrent leucocytosis, platelet consumption, fibrinogen consumption, plasminogen consumption occurring.

The non-burned tissue also has problems; these tissues swell due to increased transient vascular permeability and a decreased resistance to fluid accumulation from their low protein content.

Other considerations of stress sources to the tissue include:

1 Stress reaction/sympathetic adrenal medullary response – hormonal response of shock – the catecholamines released cause an overall hypermetabolic response: increasing body temperature, rising glucose and oxygen utilization. A catabolic or body wasting pattern will occur.

2 Immune response – is both immediate and prolonged as well as severe in nature with the presence of vasoactive amines (histamine, serotonin), complement activation, and release of prostaglandins, kinins and endotoxins occur. The overall effect is increased release of catecholamines and glucocorticoids.

The clinician needs to be cognizant of the changes not just in the areas of recognized burns but throughout

Maureen O'Reilly

the airway/respiratory system. The latter has additional concerns with exposure to chemicals, carbon monoxide and with surfactant displacement which will lead to atelectasis and respiratory distress. Burn assessment includes – reviewing the causative agent (type of burn), the extent and depth of the burn, coexistent injuries, the general health status and the patients self-care status.

Minor burn treatment includes

- Pain control.
- Cleansing the wound with non-toxic agents; copious irrigation.
- Debridement of loose tissue, broken blisters and debris, allows a better estimation of the true depth of the burn. Large intact blisters (>4–5 cm) may be left intact depending on local policy, to protect underlying dermis and decrease pain initially.

Tetanus–diphtheria immunization must be updated.

MAJOR BURN

The treatment involves hospitalization. It focuses on stopping the burning process, initiating fluid resuscitation, maintaining body core temperature and cooling the burn site. *Concurrently* the health care team initially focuses on airway, breathing and circulation adjuncts. Later the team focuses on wound management metabolic support and rehabilitation. *Airway treatment* focus' on maintaining small airway patency, removal of soot and debris and removal of mucopurulent secretions. Early intubation within 1–4 h is recommended as airway oedema will worsen after 12–18 h. PEEP is used. Bronchodilators are used to correct bronchospasm. Currently antibiotics and corticosteroids are held until needed as they can increase mortality.

The second focus in major burn treatment is *fluid resuscitation* – the goal is to maintain vascular volume, tissue perfusion and cardiac output, as well as restrict oedema formation. Initially post burn the cardiac output decreases to half, there is a return in 18–24 h to baseline. A supranormal cardiac output can occur in the acute phase of a burn. There continues to be a controversy over the use of crystalloids vs. colloids in burn care, one is referred to the recent

trauma literature for additional information. There are numerous formulas available for burn resuscitation (Evans, Brooke, Parkland, HALFD-Hypertonic Albumin-containing Fluid Demand). The Baxter-Parkland formula is most often used:

$$(4\,ml/kg \text{ of body weight}) \Big/ (\% \text{ total body surface area over } 24\,h)$$

for example $4\,ml \times 74\,kg \times 30\%$

$$4 \times 74 \times 30 = 8880\,ml$$

first 8 h from time of burn

$$\tfrac{1}{2} \text{ is administered} - 4440\,ml$$

over the next 16 h the remaining ½ is given – 2,220 ml 8 h, 2220 ml last 8 h.

In plasma leakage, the clinician often adds fresh frozen plasma infusions, with no decrease in the crystalloid administration – this has been shown to increase the hourly urine output. Urine output must be at least 30–50 ml/h in the adult and 0.7–1.0 ml/kg in children less than 30 kg.

ELECTRICAL BURNS

These are less than 2% of the burn injury population. Electrical burns are classified by voltage, type of current and length of contact. Electricity causes direct cellular de-naturation, causing healthy tissue to de-vascularize, allowing arterial and venous coagulation – overall, gross amounts of tissue is necrosed. Unlike thermal burns, with electrical burns, one cannot determine the percentage of total burn surface area. Electricity follows paths of least resistance, and has an affinity for water-containing tissue: blood and lymph vessels, nerves, well endowed organs (lungs, heart, renals, eyes, brain, etc.). It will be most resistant to the least containing water components – bone and fat. Alternating current tends to be a lower voltage increasing the likelihood of tetany, prolonging exposure to the current and causing more damage. Direct current, although most often a higher voltage, does not cause tetany.

The outcomes in an electrical burn can include: ventricular fibrillation, laryngeal spasm, respiratory arrest, seizures, coma, hypotension, retinal detachment, delayed cataract development, fractures, muscle necrosis, haemolysis of red blood cells, renal failure, haemorrhage, anaemic or other delayed neurological changes including level of consciousness, paresis or paralysis.

CHEMICAL BURNS

Chemical burns cause reactions in tissues leading to protein denaturation and heat production. Tissue destruction continues until the chemical is removed. Acids are limited by the protein present in the tissue. These include protoplasmic poisons and alkaloid acids (tannic, picric, formic, hydrofluoric, nitric and sulphuric acid).

Alkalis are more corrosive, unlimited in action, and cause deeper tissue injury. This is called tissue soponifications and desiccations. Treatment starts with removal of powders, water lavage for over 30 min or until no further chemical influence remains.

Tar can cause superficial to deep/full thickness burns. Avoid hydrocarbon solvents during the removal process; mineral oil is most frequently used.

Bibliography

Alexander R, Proctor H, eds (1995) *Advanced trauma life support course*. American College of Surgeons, Publishers.

Bayfront Medical Center (1988) *Trauma nurse specialist: program manual*. St Petersburg, Florida: Bayfront Medical Center.

Bayley E, Turcke SA (1992) *A comprehensive curriculum for trauma nursing*. Jones and Bartlett.

Bronson Methodist Hospital (1990) *Trauma nursing course*. Kalamazoo, Michigan: Bronson Methodist Hospital.

Cardona V, Hurn P, Mason PJ, Scanlon-Schilpp A, Veise-Berry S (1988) *Trauma nursing: from resuscitation to rehabilitation*. London: W.B. Saunders.

Dolan B, Holt L (2000) *Accident and emergency theory into practice* London: Bailliere Tindal.

Dunham CM, Crowley RA (1991) *Shock trauma critical care manual: maryland institute of emergency medical services system*. Aspen.

Emergency Nurses Association (1994) *Emergency nursing core curriculum*, 4th ed. London: W.B. Saunders.

Featherstone K, Hilton G, Jastremski CW (1998) *Instructors resource manual for trauma nursing*. W.B. Saunders.

Hodgetts T, Deane S, Gunning K (1997) *Trauma rules*. BMJ Publishing Group.

Holleran RS (1994). *Prehospital nursing: a collaborative approach*. Mosby.

Joy C (1989) *Paediatric trauma nursing*. Aspen.

Knezevich B (1986) *Trauma nursing: principles and practice*. Appleton-Century-Crofts.

Markovchick V, Pons P, Wolfe R (1993) *Emergency medicine secrets*. Hanley and Belfus.

Nef J, Kidd PS (1993) *Trauma nursing: the art and science*. Mosby.

Oman K, Koziol-McLain J, Scheetz L (2001) *Emergency nursing secrets*. Hanley and Belfus.

O'Reilly, Maureen (2001) *Trauma nursing course: St Barnabas Medical Centre Program*. St Barnabas Medical Center.

Rea R, ed. (1991) *Trauma nurse core course* 3rd ed. Emergency Nurses Association, Award Publishing Corporation.

Sheehy SB (1991) *Emergency nursing: principle and practice*. 3rd ed. London: Mosby.

Sheehy SB (1994) *Manual of clinical trauma care: the first hour* 2nd ed. London: Mosby.

Welton R, Shane K, eds (1990) *Case studies in trauma nursing*. Williams and Wilkins.

8 | Emergency care of the person with minor injury and minor illness

Gary Jones

This chapter focuses on assessing, diagnosing and managing minor injuries/illness that in many settings are now managed exclusively by nurses. Minor head, eye, ear, nose, throat and limb injuries are addressed, together with management of wounds and infections. Whilst recommended treatments are included, these will differ in some units therefore the emphasis is on assessment, which is key to the diagnosis.

INTRODUCTION

The term minor injury or minor illness continues to be debated. What is considered minor to one person may be considered major to another. In many cases (e.g. head injury) the term "minor" can only be used once a full assessment/examination has been undertaken and no abnormality identified. With the introduction of nurse led minor injury units, walk in centres, NHS Direct and fast track minor injury/illness services within Emergency Departments many people now identify what they perceive as "minor" and either attend such units or telephone for advice.

When nurse led services became more popular and minor injury units became more available during the late 1980s and throughout the 1990s, great debate ensued as to the public's ability to determine what constituted a minor injury. Dale and Dolan (1996) identified the lack of agreement on what constitutes a minor injury unit in terms of the basic range of services. They identify "concern has been voiced,

particularly by some members of the Emergency Department profession, that patients may misjudge their needs and so inadvertently delay receiving care requiring specialist skills and resources".

While these concerns remain, a number of studies have shown that patients do choose appropriately (Jones 1993; Dale and Dolan 1996; Heaney 1997; Paxton 1997). Therefore nurses will continue to develop services that are focused on the provision of minor injury/illness care and within the context of ensuring that the nursing assessment, diagnosis, intervention and final decision regarding discharge or referral is based on a sound knowledge base.

DETERMINING A MINOR INJURY/ILLNESS

When confronted with a patient, who is complaining of what appears to be a minor injury or illness, it is essential that the nurse uses a structured approach to the assessment, diagnosis, intervention and evaluation.

While the overall approach to patient care should include using the framework discussed in Chapter 2, the very nature of the nurse moving to a diagnosis and prescribing treatment without the input from medical staff requires the nurse to have additional examination skills. History and mechanism of injury or illness remains the key. The assessment and examination will involve new skills such as percussion and auscultation. Most importantly it will involve having the ability to consider differential diagnosis and from the examination rule out those that do not apply and consider those that do. Three possibilities

Emergency care of the person with minor injury and minor illness

emerge:

Confident with diagnosis minor injury/illness	Uncertain diagnosis	Confident with diagnosis not a minor injury/illness
↓	↓	↓
Treat and discharge	Refer	Refer

In the majority of cases minor injury or illness normally requires the nurse to focus on a specific problem and usually a specific area of the body. In fact in many units minor injury/illness is defined as:

- Minor head and neck injury with no loss of consciousness
- Eye emergencies including superficial foreign bodies in the eye, superficial infections of lids and conjunctiva
- Ear, nose and throat problems including foreign bodies in the nose and epistaxis, foreign bodies in the ear
- Limb injuries/conditions usually below elbow or below knee
- Wounds including superficial wounds, burns and scalds, stings and small bites
- Coughs, colds, high temperatures, skin rashes.

While units will differ in the range of conditions the nurse is allowed to treat the underlying principles of patient care must remain. It is essential that the nurse:

- Obtains a full history of the event including the mechanism of injury
- Undertakes a full assessment of the patient and the specific area of injury/complaint
- Uses investigations such as X-ray when appropriate
- Determines the diagnosis
- Provides treatment
- Determines the need for referral or discharge
- Provides self-care advice and follow-up as necessary.

HEAD INJURY

Minor head injury applies to those patients who are fully orientated, have amnesia of less than 10 min,

have no neurological signs or symptoms at the time of the examination and have no skull fracture (Driscoll et al 1993).

Head injuries can be classified under three anatomical sites: the scalp, the skull and the brain (Dawson and Sanders 2000).

Scalp injuries can range from simple bruising to large wounds. Skull fractures occur at the point of impact and can be linear or depressed. In major trauma the skull may be fractured into multiple fragments (comminuted).

The brain is poorly anchored within the skull; it is liable to move within the skull in response to acceleration or deceleration. Contact between the surface of the brain and the interior skull causes bruising. Internal shearing forces leads to stretching and tearing of brain tissue. Mild stretching leads to transient disturbance of consciousness know as concussion.

Concussion

A transient form of diffuse injury resulting in minor head injury. It is graded into four severity groups:

- Grade 1: No loss of consciousness, transient confusion and rapid return to normal function
- Grade 2: Confusion and mild amnesia
- Grade 3: Profound confusion and pre- and post-amnesia
- Grade 4: Loss of consciousness, variable confusion, and amnesia.
                              (Dawson and Sanders 2000)

Assessment

One of the most essential aspects of the assessment is to determine if the patient is suffering from a minor head injury or a significant injury that requires referral.

History
- What was the mechanism of injury?
  Establish the speed of impact, nature of object that struck the head, part of the head involved and area of contact (e.g. occipital area hitting a carpeted floor is less serious than the temple hitting the corner of a table or a football boot striking the temple area of the skull).

- What is the patient complaining of? Headache, nausea and vomiting may be normal responses to a bump on the head but if reoccurring can be early signs of raised intracranial pressure.
- Was there any loss of consciousness? How long? History of altered consciousness is an indication for skull X-ray (Moulton and Yates 1999) and linked with other features may suggest the need for admission to hospital. Young children lose consciousness less readily than adults do. Significant brain injury may occur without a history of unconsciousness.
- Establish what recollection of events both pre- and post-injury the patient has?
- Any drugs or alcohol involved? These may be the cause of the altered conscious state.
- Any history of fits? Now or in the past?

Neurological assessment – determine the patient's neurological status

The most important aspect of the assessment of any head-injured patient is altered level of consciousness and the duration of post-traumatic amnesia.

- Assess the conscious state. Start by using the AVPU tool
- Move on to a formal Glasgow Coma Scale (GCS)
- Record:
  - Blood pressure
  - Pulse
  - Respiration rate and quality
  - Temperature
  - Pupil reaction
  - Limb movements.

By taking all of the recordings together a reasonably accurate picture of the patient's condition can be obtained.

Changes in the neurological score are very significant and will often indicate signs of deterioration well before any other parameter changes.

The results of the GCS score can be classified into three groups (Dawson and Sanders 2000):

- Scores 13–15 indicative of a minor head injury
- Scores 9–12 suggest moderate head injury or a more severe head injury beginning to be demonstrated
- Score 8 or less suggests severe head injury.

Scalp and skull

The scalp should be assessed for any wounds, bruising, boggy areas and tenderness. Wounds should be cleaned and examined for any foreign bodies. Caution should be exercised when exploring the wound if glass is suspected as a foreign body. The wound should be palpated with a gloved finger to detect any fracture lines (except if glass is suspected).

Indications for skull X-ray

Suspected penetrating injury, any alteration in neurological status, significant bruising or swelling to the scalp, high speed injury to the temporal and parietal areas of the skull are all indicators for skull X-ray. Moulton and Yates (1999), Howarth and Evans (1994) also advocate skull X-ray in any patient with a history of altered consciousness or amnesia at any time. Moulton and Yates (1999) also advocate X-rays if the patient has vomited even once.

Intervention for scalp wounds will depend on the extent of injury but normally require either suturing, staples or glue.

Refer or discharge?

The risk of developing any complications from a head injury is influenced by a number of factors:

1 The level of consciousness: Most references appear to base the risk not so much on the period of unconsciousness prior to arrival but more on the conscious level at the time of presentation. However Moulton and Yates (1999) suggest that patients who are fully alert on examination but with a history of an altered level of consciousness before arrival have a higher risk of developing complications. An impaired level of consciousness

at the time of presentation has a risk of complications of 1 in 180 compared to 1 in 8000 in those who are fully conscious.

2 Post-traumatic amnesia: More than 15 min duration increases the risk of complications.

3 Neurological abnormalities, fits, severe headaches, persistent vomiting and skull fractures all increase the risk of complications.

Discharge should only occur if the patient has suffered a minor head injury. All other patients should be referred for probable admission. The decision must be based on the following criteria:

- Fully conscious on presentation
- No abnormal neurological signs
- Loss of consciousness or post-traumatic amnesia of less than 5 min
- No severe headache or vomiting
- No skull fracture
- No bleeding disorder
- Good home conditions (i.e. support/not alone)
- Reliable relative or friend available to take the patient home and maintain head injury observations.

(Moulton and Yates 1999)

The relative or friend should be instructed to observe the individual hourly then 2 hourly for 24 h. Ensure the individual remains alert to time and place and returns/attends an Emergency Department if there is any deterioration, drowsiness, confusion, severe headaches, vomiting, weakness or fits, fluid or blood from the ears. Analgesia if required should be paracetamol for general aches/pains but not used for increasing headache.

NECK INJURY

Like head injury, a neck injury can only be termed minor once a full assessment has been carried out. Many patients will attend Emergency Departments, Minor Injury Units or walk in centres with neck pain. The majority will have occurred from a "whiplash" of the neck following a road traffic incident. A "stiff

neck" with no history of trauma is another such common complaint.

Attendance at the minor injuries/illness service normally suggests that the patient is alert and able to provide the history and mechanism of injury. The mechanism of injury is essential and will allow the nurse to determine if the neck injury is significant and requires cervical/spinal immobilization or can be treated and the patient discharged home.

WHIPLASH ASSOCIATED DISORDER

Whiplash is a common, disabling condition associated with an acceleration–deceleration mechanism of energy transfer. It is commonly a result of rear or side impact motor vehicle accidents, but can also be caused by sport. Whiplash is a diagnosis that can only be made after a thorough examination. The forces involved can cause bony injury or soft tissue injuries (whiplash) leading to clinical manifestations such as neurological symptoms (whiplash associated disorder). Assessing an individual with neck pain and deciding whether a C-spine radiography is required is often challenging. Hoffman et al (2000) have identified five criteria that, if met, suggest that the individual has a very low likelihood of C-spine injury. These criteria have been developed into an acronym, to assist clinicians in determining the likelihood of C-spine injury and therefore the need for C-spine imaging. This acronym is presented in the box below and has an extra component added, safe movement, and is used by nurses to clinically clear C-spine injuries. If the criteria devised by Hoffman et al (2000) are utilized (i.e. the answers to the questions are negative) then under the right clinical circumstances the individual may not require C-spine radiographs (Vinson 2001).

Assessment

Neurological examination: any focal deficit?
Spine examination: any tenderness in the posterior midline of the cervical spine?
Alertness: any alteration to level of consciousness or orientation?
Intoxication: any evidence of drugs or alcohol?
Distracting injury: any painful injury that might distract the patient from the pain of a cervical spine injury?

Safe movement: is there any pain on movement (lateral rotation, lateral flexion, flexion/extension)? (Adapted by Crouch 2001, from Vinson 2001)

Treatment

Exercise: Encourage the person to move their neck and return to normal activities as soon as possible. Perform gentle and slow neck exercises during the first few days. These include turning the head slowly from side to side as if looking over their shoulder; slowly moving their left ear down to their left shoulder then doing the same with their right and lastly moving their chin towards their chest and then looking up towards the ceiling. These exercises should be repeated about six times a day. The patient should be advised not to continue if they have excessive pain or dizziness, and they should not circle their head and neck. This may be a little painful, but this should ease.

Analgesia: the drugs of choice are non-steroidal anti-inflammatories (as long as no contraindications).

Sleeping: they should be advised to try and keep their neck straight when sleeping on their side.

Stiff neck

The most common cause of stiff neck (Torticollis or Wryneck) is abnormal positioning of the neck muscles. Local spasm occurs in one of the sternomastoid muscles. The patient will normally complain of severe pain and spasm of the effected muscle. There is no history of trauma.

> **Assessment and Treatment**
> - Local tenderness, restricted movement especially rotation.
> - Analgesia and a local non-steroidal cream and gentle manipulation often helps (Moulton and Yates 1999).

EYE EMERGENCIES

The eye can either be damaged through infection/inflammation or trauma. Both blunt and penetrating trauma can seriously damage the eye.

Assessment

> **History/mechanism**
> - What is the complaint?
> - Any foreign body – low or high velocity? Foreign bodies that blow into the eye are normally low velocity. Those from grinding stones, chipping at stone are normally high velocity.
> - Identify if the patient is photophobic? If looking at light causes pain then the patient is photophobic until proven otherwise. This suggests intra-ocular inflammation and referral is appropriate.
> - Is the patient complaining of pain?
> - Has there been any bleeding/discharge? Irritation and discharge suggest superficial problems. Pain or an ache suggests intra-ocular problems.

Visual acuity

Visual acuity means the acuteness of sight, in other words how well you can see. The distant visual acuity is tested using a Snellen's eye test chart. Visual acuity should be recorded before any intervention (excluding the administration of anaesthetic drops or eye irrigation for burns/chemicals). It provides a base line from which to work and also affords some legal protection.

The Snellen chart must be 6 m from the patient. If distance is a problem then 3 m charts are available. As well as the standard letters charts, E charts or charts with symbols such as children's toys should make it possible to test the visual acuity of most patients.

When testing the patients vision stand the patient 6 m from the standard chart, cover one eye. Record the line read. When recording the vision on the record chart, always record the distance that the patient stands away from the chart above the line read, e.g. 6/6 or 6/60 (Figure 8.1). If the patient reads most of a line but cannot clearly see one or two letters, then this is recorded as 6/the line number minus the number of letters missed, e.g. 6/9 − 2. If only one or two letters in a line are read, then the line above is recorded but with a plus for the letters read on the

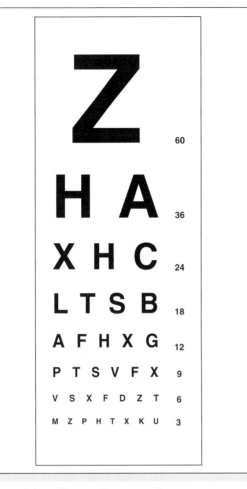

Z	60
H A	36
X H C	24
L T S B	18
A F H X G	12
P T S V F X	9
V S X F D Z T	6
M Z P H T X K U	3

Figure 8.1 Snellen visual acuity eye chart

Clinical assessment

Once the history has been obtained and the visual acuity recorded, the nurse is now ready to clinically assess the patients' eye. *Some general principles need to be considered before the assessment begins.*

The eye or eyes can become red due to a number of causes. While simple superficial infections or foreign bodies cause most of the red eyes that are treated in the minor injury setting, it is essential not to become overconfident. *Always put together the history, visual acuity and the eye examination.* A number of patients have been treated incorrectly for conjunctivitis when the condition was iritis.

Apart from inflammatory disorders where the visual acuity can become diminished or lost, or trauma related conditions that can affect vision, other conditions that can cause partial or total loss of vision can include retinal detachment, retinal artery occlusion, optic nerve ischaemia or retinal vein occlusion. *Any sudden loss or diminished visual acuity, with or without pain must be treated as an ophthalmic emergency.*

When assessing always assess both eyes and compare both eyes.

Use a good bright light. Identify if the light causes pain. Chong and Murray (1993) found that a simple test with a pen torch might help distinguish between mild and serious ocular problems in patients with unilateral red eye. From a distance of 15 cm, a light shone for 2 seconds into the affected eye gave a positive increase in discomfort in 68% of patients suffering with iritis. This compared with no positive results in the unaffected eye. Use of a slit lamp will give a magnified view of the eye as well as providing depth perception. The ophthalmoscope allows for visual access beyond the pupil.

X-ray may be indicated if an intra-ocular foreign body is suspected. X-rays do not always show up foreign bodies and ultrasound is more helpful (McElvanney and Fielder 1993).

As part of the routine assessment of the eye always stain the eye with fluorescein. Fluorescein sodium is used to detect lesions most commonly those of the cornea. Any damage to the corneal tissue will become stained with the fluorescein and a green area will be seen. The fluorescein can be quite concentrated and the use of a normal saline drop after the installation of the

next line down, e.g. 6/12 + 2. If the patient cannot see 6/60 move them forward each metre, e.g. 3/60. If the patient is unable to see the top letter (60), test if they can see and count fingers, identify hand movements or finally distinguish light and dark. If spectacles for distant vision are used, always ask the patient to wear these when you are testing the visual acuity, but remember to record that spectacles were used. Always test both eyes and record your findings. The use of pinholes (a small hole in a piece of card or plastic) does allow a more accurate visual acuity to be obtained in patients with a poor vision. Pinholes are useful if the patient normally wears spectacles for distance vision but these are not available or have been broken.

fluorescein can sometimes result in a much better stain. Routine use of fluorescein as part of the eye examination should be encouraged (excluding penetrating injuries). This is especially important when the patient gives a history of possible foreign body entering the eye or any injury to the eye that may have caused a corneal abrasion. Ensure the patient has removed any soft contact lenses before instilling. Soft contact lenses take up the stain and become damaged beyond repair. Prior to the patient's discharge, good practice also includes washing the stain out of the eye.

A number of old wives tales still exist regarding the use of and length of time anaesthetic drops remain active. In the minor injury setting the two most widely used topical anaesthetics are amethocaine hydrochloride and oxybuprocaine hydrochloride (Benoxinate). All topical anaesthetics can cause delayed healing and epithelial defects to the cornea; this is why patients should not be given such drugs to instil regularly. Although one drug may be more irritant than another, the toxicity to corneal epithelium and the length of activity makes cocaine an unpopular drug for routine use (BNF 1999). Cocaine has an effect of some 4–6 h and it is this that still leads many people to believe all topical anaesthetics have a similar action. In reality amethocaine and benoxinate, especially in the low doses used in Emergency Department, have short life spans lasting some 20–30 min, and therefore the use of eye pads are often unnecessary and in many departments are grossly over used.

Examination of structures

The examination should be conducted in a logical journey from the lids to the conjunctiva, then to the cornea, anterior chamber, iris and pupil. The lens will be seen if a cataract is present. The inside of the eye including the retina can be seen using an ophthalmoscope. Inspect the globe for any damage. Check the tension of the eye by gently palpating both eyes with your fingers (rule out ocular damage first). A soft eye may indicate a fluid leak. A hard eye can be due to glaucoma. Check eye movements.

Even if you discover a problem, continue your journey so that you do not miss any other problem. At the end of your journey, identify what problems you have found and treat or refer.

The general principles that will help distinguish a minor eye condition from a more serious complaint can often be determined from the history and visual acuity.

- Low velocity foreign bodies usually suggest superficial injury.
- High velocity usually suggests intra-ocular injury.
- An itchy, sticky, watery eye normally suggests superficial problems.
- Superficial pain (linked with history of trauma) usually suggests superficial injury.
- Aching, painful eyes, photophobia and/or visual changes usually suggests intra-ocular problems.

Lids

Assess overall condition including the eyelashes. Lacerations should be referred unless superficial. Bruising and swelling (having ruled out any underlying damage) respond well to cold compress and ice packs. Antibiotic ointment will normally treat most infections.

Blepharitis

Cause	Bacterial infection of the lid margins
Appearance	Lids become red, puffy, sticky
Treatment	Antibiotic ointment rubbed onto the eyelid margins
Advice	Regarding cross infection

Stye

Cause	Bacterial infection of the hair follicle
Appearance	Small infected area on the lid margin at the hair follicle
Treatment	Antibiotic ointment
Advice	Regarding cross infection

Conjunctiva

The conjunctiva should be transparent. Redness of the conjunctiva (the red eye) can be due to superficial infection or intra-ocular inflammation. Always ensure your assessment does not confuse one for the other.

Conjunctivitis

Cause	Viral or bacterial infection
Appearance	Sore watery eyes or gritty sticky eyes (unilateral or bilateral). Redness of the conjunctiva is often distributed across the conjunctiva but more acute towards the periphery. Do not confuse with iritis (see iritis)
Treatment	Antibiotic drops and ointment if bacterial Artificial tears if viral

Allergic conjunctivitis

Cause	Reaction to usually pollen or dust entering the eye
Appearance	The conjunctiva becomes oedematous, the eye(s) water and become itchy
Treatment	Antihistamine locally or systemically
Advice	Advice that the oedema will subside. No further treatment is normally required

Sub-conjunctival bleeds

Cause	Trauma or spontaneous. If spontaneous usually associated with an increased pressure or underlying medical condition (cough, vomiting, hypertension, and diabetes)
Appearance	Area of blood under the conjunctiva
Treatment	Ensure other injury or medical condition is ruled out (check blood pressure and urine for sugar). No treatment required
Advice	Advise and reassure the patient that the blood will disappear over the next few days. Changes in colour are normal

Sub-tarsal foreign body

Cause	Foreign body blown into the eye and it becomes stuck on the sub-tarsal plate
Appearance	When the eyelid is everted the foreign body can be seen
Treatment	Removal using a moist cotton bud. Stain the cornea to identify any abrasion. If no abrasion then no further treatment is required
Advice	Dependent on the cause and may include use of protective glasses

Cornea

The cornea is the window of the eye. It should be crystal clear. White rings around the periphery of the cornea are of no significance in the elderly but can be a sign of a metabolic disorder in the young.

When assessing the cornea with a light source, a good reflection of the light should be obtained.

Corneal foreign bodies and abrasions

Cause	Foreign bodies blow onto the cornea. An object scratching the cornea including fingers, edges of papers flicked into the eye, will cause abrasions
Appearance	Foreign bodies will be seen. Abrasions will be identified with the use of fluorescein stain
Treatment	Local anaesthetic. Remove the foreign body. Antibiotic ointment. A pad can help the healing in some cases
Advice	May include use of protective glasses

Arc eye

Cause	Ultraviolet light usually from arc welding or a sunbed
Appearance	Red, watery, photophobic, very painful eyes

Treatment	Local anaesthetic. Simple lubricant (liquid paraffin or non-antibiotic ointment). Regular systemic analgesia
Advice	Rest in darkened room. Sunglasses for 24–36 h. Use of protective glasses in the future

Anterior chamber

The anterior chamber lies between the back of the cornea and the iris. It contains aqueous humour. The chamber can become damaged or more commonly blood from damage to the iris vessels can be seen inside the chamber (hyphaema). A patient with a hyphaema should be referred to the ophthalmic services ensuring the person remains resting in a semi-recumbent position.

Glaucoma (increased pressure within the globe) can also occur. The patient will experience severe pain in the eye and diminished vision. This condition requires urgent referral.

Iris

The iris allows light through the pupil and can become inflamed normally due to a systemic problem such as rheumatoid arthritis, systemic lupus or a range of other autoimmune type conditions.

This condition can sometimes be confused with conjunctivitis and results in incorrect treatment being prescribed.

Iritis

Cause	Systemic inflammatory conditions
Appearance	Red conjunctiva normally unilateral (often more acute around the cornea and less towards the periphery). Slight diminished vision. Photophobia. Pupil may be irregularly shaped. Ache/pain in the eye
Treatment	Refer to ophthalmic unit

Other eye conditions

These conditions include burns, perforation of the globe, retinal detachment and injuries to the orbit. They all require referral to the ophthalmic unit.

EAR, NOSE AND THROAT CONDITIONS
Epistaxis

This condition is often spontaneous in children and occurs from Little's area on the anterior part of the septum. Precipitating causes are allergic rhinitis or minor trauma secondary to picking their nose.

In adults, bleeding usually occurs further back and is commonly associated with hypertension. It may also occur in patients taking anticoagulants.

In the elderly, bleeding commonly occurs high in the posterior part of the nose due to damage to other atherosclerotic vessels and can bleed profusely leading to hypovolaemic shock.

Intervention

- Apply pressure to the anterior part of the nose for approximately 10 min with the patient sitting upwards and forwards (Howarth and Evans 1994).
- Once the bleeding has stopped, the patient should be advised not to pick or blow their nose and to avoid hot drinks or spicy foods for at least 24 h.
- If the bleeding persists remove any clot, identify the affected area and refer.

Nasal foreign bodies

- An attempt can be made using a pair of Tilly's forceps to remove the object if easily visualized.
- Spherical objects are often difficult to grasp and it may be necessary to use low-pressure suction to try and dislodge these.
- It is not advisable to attempt removal more than once or twice before referring to the ENT department.

Foreign bodies in the ear

- Removal may be achieved using aural forceps.
- If an insect is removed, it is especially important to check the canal for debris or eggs. It is also

important that the patient is given information regarding signs and symptoms of infection and told to attend their GP should this occur.

Bleeding tooth socket

- Identify the area of bleeding.
- Place a gauze roll into the socket.
- Encourage the patient to bite onto a pad placed on the gauze roll.

Swallowed foreign bodies

- Treatment will depend on the item swallowed. Often smooth non-toxic items will cause no problems and no treatment is required.
- Seek advise as necessary from the regional poison's unit.

LIMB INJURIES/NON-TRAUMATIC CONDITIONS

The vast majority of minor limb injuries include wounds, burns and scalds and musculo-skeletal injuries (usually but not exclusively below the elbow or knee). Non-traumatic conditions often include inflammatory disorders, gout or localized infection.

Musculo-skeletal injuries

Musculo-skeletal problems account for an estimated 3.5 million Emergency Department attendances each year. Many of these are self-limiting conditions such as bruises and sprains, which will often only require simple advice (Wardrope and English 1998).

> ### Assessment
> - History.
> - Mechanism of injury.
> - Inspect the skin for injury or any changes in colour. Look at the shape of the limb for any swelling or deformity. Compare the affected limb or area to the unaffected side. Although gross areas of swelling and bruising may be obvious, subtle areas of swelling or deformity will be missed unless a direct comparison is made.
> - Proceed to palpate in a logical manner following a specific pattern.

> Commence palpation at a joint proximal to the area of injury. Keep a careful watch on the patient's face for signs of pain whilst examining the injury.
> - Ask the patient to move (active movement) the joint before you move it (passive movement). This will give you an idea of the range of movement and whether it is painful or not. Active and passive movements test the joint function, resisted movement assesses the muscles and tendons and stress testing assesses the ligaments.
> - Assess the five Ps
>   - Pain
>   - Pallor
>   - Pulses (distal to the injury)
>   - Paresthesia (any loss of sensation)
>   - Paralysis (any loss of movement distal to the injury).
> - Following examination of the injury – X-ray may be requested.

SPRAINS AND STRAINS
Sprains

Sprains involve injury to ligaments. Normally when the ligament is stretched the protective muscle reflexes are activated. If the force is so great or if so suddenly applied that no other protective reflex is possible then the ligament will take the full effect of the force and it will tear. Ligament damage can result in a tear of a few fibres up to complete rupture of a whole ligament.

Although any ligament can be injured, the most common joint is the ankle. Ankle injuries account for 5% of the workload of an average Emergency Department (Wardrope and English 1998). Most of these injuries will be partial sprains of the anterior talofibular ligament. Other ligaments involved include the calcaneal fibular ligament and the posterior talofibular ligament.

Examination of the ankle needs to include the proximal fibula, which can be injured in severe ankle ligament injuries. The decision to X-ray should be based on the "Ottawa Ankle Rules" or at least have these included in local protocols.

Ottawa Ankle Rules – X-ray if the patient
- Is unable to weight bear immediately post injury or in the department
- Has bony tenderness over the posterior aspects of the lateral or medial malleolus
- Pain on palpation of the proximal fibula
- Specific tenderness of calcaneus, navicular or base of 5th metatarsal

Additional local criteria may also include
- Is over 55 years
- Has marked ankle swelling
- Has pain at the tip of the distal fibula
- Is unable to walk four steps in the department

Treatment of a sprain depends on the degree of injury. Classification of these injuries is as follows:

Grade 1: Minor sprain

There is stretching of the ligament without macroscopic tearing of the ligament. It is characterized by minor/moderate mechanism of injury, some disability, moderate localized swelling and tenderness.

Treatment is based on the RICE principle.

Rest initially to help pain and overcome swelling.
Ice for 10 min, 3–4 times per day (applied over a cloth to prevent burns).
Compression to avoid swelling.
Elevation of the limb above the heart.

In addition to the above – rehabilitation as soon as possible to allow early return to full function and analgesia are advised.

Grade 2: Moderate sprain

There is partial macroscopic tearing of the ligament characterized by significant mechanism of injury, moderate swelling, pain and often the patient is partial weight bearing.

Treatment principles are the same as for a minor sprain, but often crutches are required and the patient may need to be reviewed, either in the Emergency Department or the fracture clinic. Physiotherapy may be indicated for those patients with high functional demands or who require an early return to work or sport.

Grade 3: Severe sprain

Involves complete rupture of the ligament. Characterized by significant mechanism of injury, massive swelling, unable to weight bear, signs of instability.

Initial treatment may consist of advice to elevate the limb, apply a back slab of plaster of Paris and to give crutches and analgesia. Surgical repair can sometimes be necessary to treat this type of injury.

Controversy still exists regarding compression. Watts and Armstrong (2001) indicate that there is no well conducted randomized controlled trials on the optimum treatment for grade 1 and 2 ankle sprains. Their trial comparing no compression with the use of double tubigrip concluded that treatment of grade 1 and 2 ankle sprains with double tubigrip does not seem to lead to a shorter time to functional recovery and may increase the requirement for analgesia. They recognize that other complex wraps, braces or intensive rehabilitation programmes have been studied.

Local protocols will vary on the methods (or not) of compression; with some favouring elastoplast strapping and others using a variety of other support methods.

Strains

Strains occur when the muscle fibres or tendons are stretched beyond the normal length. Common areas include the Gastrocnemius muscles in the back of the lower leg and the tendon of Achilles although muscles in the arms, upper leg and the torso muscles are all vulnerable when stretched beyond normal use.

Like sprains, strains can be classified under grade (degree) and treatment is very similar.

Pulled elbow

This usually occurs in children under the age of 5.

History and mechanism of injury
- A pulling of the arm usually by the parent lifting the child by the arms
- The child will not use the arm
- The radial head (which is poorly formed at this age) has slipped through the annular ligament at the elbow.

Treatment
- Reduction is usually straight forward and the child immediately uses the arm normally
- An X-ray is not normally indicated unless there is any suspicion of a bony injury (Moulton and Yates 1999).

FRACTURES

Some minor injury services allow the initial treatment of undisplaced fractures of lower arm, hands, fingers, fibula, foot and toes where a full examination has shown no signs or symptoms of vascular or neurological damage. The patient must be referred to the local fracture clinic for on going care. Fracture of the clavicle can also be treated and referred to fracture clinic.

Forearm, wrist

Falls onto the outstretched hand may transmit forces up the entire limb and can result in a variety of injuries including fracture of the clavicle.

Common fractures and treatment
- Distal radius and ulna fracture – Plaster of Paris backslab or cast
- Scaphoid fracture – Scaphoid cast
- Colles fracture – Backslab or Colles cast.

All fractures are normally referred to the local fracture clinic. All patients must be given self-care instructions especially relating to care of the plaster cast and observations to be made regarding local vascular and neurological symptoms.

Hand, fingers

History is of specific importance particularly in the case of "punch injuries" and the resulting presence of a wound. Always think "Human Bite" and question the patient accordingly.

When assessing the thumb/fingers it is essential to name not number, therefore use thumb, index, middle, ring, little. The borders of the fingers are described as radial or ulna and the hand surfaces are described as dorsal or palmar (volar). Examine the extensor tendons, flexor tendons, and collateral ligaments.

Fractures of the distal phalanx (often secondary to a crush injury) middle phalanx and proximal phalanx are common injuries. Hand fractures (metacarpals) will depend on the mechanism of injury. Fracture of the metacarpal neck is often termed the boxer's fracture and results from punch injuries.

Treatment of fractures to the metacarpals and phalanges is with use of neighbour strapping/support bandage. A mallet splint is required for mallet deformity or fracture to the distal interphalangeal joint.

Prophylactic antibiotics are required for any human or animal bite.

Common non-traumatic conditions and treatment
- Paronychia – requires dressing, possible drainage and antibiotics
- Herpetic whitlow – requires antiviral treatment
- Pulp space infection – requires antibiotics and referral.

FOOT AND ANKLE INJURIES (BELOW KNEE)
Ankle

The majority of ankle injuries will be sprains. However always consider strain or rupture injury to the Achilles tendon. Fracture of the calcaneum should also be considered when examining an ankle injury.

Common fractures of the ankle include:

- distal fibula
- avulsion of lateral malleolus
- avulsion of talus
- avulsion of cuboid
- medial malleolus
- navicular.

Treatment of these fractures often requires support strapping and in some instances may require a below knee cast.

Foot, toes

A common injury to the foot includes a fracture of the base of the 5th metatarsal due to an inversion injury.

A stubbed toe injury is another common presentation in minor injuries units. Fractures of the great toe may require the patient to be non-weight bearing and subsequently referred to the fracture clinic. Other toe fractures can be X-rayed according to local policy and treated with neighbour strapping.

Non-traumatic conditions of the toe can include:

- paronychia – requires dressing, possible drainage and antibiotics;
- ingrown toe nail – local treatment including possible wedge resection.

WOUNDS

The skin can become injured by a number of mechanisms and the management of the wound will often depend on the mechanism of injury.

Mechanical mechanism of injury

Mechanical injuries to the skin are very common and are caused by items such as sharp blades, wire, metal, and bullets. This mechanism of injury causes a variety of wounds including:

- Incised wound – clean cut such as with a knife.
- Laceration – irregular cuts such as from barbed wire.
- Abrasion – superficial removal of skin such as rubbing on a hard surface.
- Bleeding varicose veins – often a small knock will cause a varicose vein to bleed profusely and yet hardly any wound will be seen.
- Puncture wound – a small hole penetrating the skin. Remember it may be deep and cause internal damage.
- Gunshot wound – this may cause a small entry site and large exit wound.
- Crush injury – this is where the tissue is squashed.
- Amputation – a part of a limb completely severed from the body.

All wounds may have underlying muscle, tendon, nerve, blood vessel or bone damage. Internal structures (especially the gut in an abdominal wound) can protrude from the wound.

Puncture wounds can be caused by sharp instruments or from snakes and insects.

Gunshot wounds can cause a range of damage dependant on the velocity of the bullet. Low velocity bullets create a track while high velocity bullets can create massive cavities and internal damage due to the released energy.

Crush injuries release toxic waste (myloglobin), which can affect the kidneys and lungs.

From a treatment standpoint there are essentially two types of wounds: those, which are characterized by loss of tissue and those in which no tissue has been lost (Westaby 1985).

Thermal injuries to the skin are of two types

- *Burns* caused by dry heat, chemicals, friction, electricity, ultraviolet light and radiation
- *Scalds* caused by wet heat, the commonest being hot liquids and vapours.

The surface area that is injured and the depth of the burn determine the severity of a burn or scald.

Burn depth is identified as

- Superficial – redness, swelling and painful.
- Partial thickness – very red, blisters and/or some skin loss. Painful.
- Full thickness – Pale or black, the skin appears like leather. No pain.

Where full thickness burns have occurred there will normally be areas of partial thickness and superficial injury creating a mixed wound.

Infection

All wounds are effectively contaminated because the normal integrity of the skin has been breached and therefore infection is always possible. The degree of contamination will often determine the risk.

Tetanus is of particular concern especially in wounds that are deep (puncture wounds) although all wounds may be contaminated with tetanus. Tetanus toxoid prevents tetanus but if the patient has never been immunized or there is a high risk of contamination tetanus immunoglobulin should be administered.

Assessment/examination of the wound

The key to the treatment of minor wounds, burns and scalds lies in the assessment.

Before any decision can be made as to the best treatment for a wound a number of factors need to be considered:

- Mechanism of injury. What caused the wound? Does the mechanism suggest possible underlying damage to nerves, blood vessels, tendons, bone, etc.?
- Time of injury – wounds more than 6 h old are more likely to get infected (Moulton and Yates 1999).
- Place of injury – garden?
- Tetanus status.
- Location of the wound.
- On general examination is there any loss of function/sensation in the area of injury/distal to the injury? Any circulatory problems distal to the injury?
- If a burn/scald – the amount of surface area affected and depth.

Patients who present with an acute tissue inflammation/infection should have an urinalysis/BM stick performed as well as temperature recorded.

Inspecting the wound
Carefully inspect the wound. Use local anaesthetic if necessary.
- Degree of bleeding – type of bleeding
  - Capillary bleeding oozes from the wound
  - Venous bleeding flows from the wound
  - Arterial bleeding spurts from the wound.
- Assess the depth, type, site, length and width of the wound.
- Check for any contamination/foreign bodies. X-ray for radio-opaque foreign bodies may be required (Howarth and Evans 1994).
- Tissue viability.
- Tissue loss.

Treatment – helping the natural healing processes

Wounds can either be closed or allowed to heal with or without a dressing. Closure of a wound is achieved using adhesive skin closures, glue, staples or sutures.

Wound dressings are numerous and the type of dressing will be determined by the assessment of the wound and local guidelines.

Before closing or dressing a wound the wound must be cleaned and foreign bodies removed (unless embedded deep in the wound). In some cases this may require local anaesthetic. Digital nerve blocks are very effective if providing a little anaesthesia when dealing with finger injuries.

The exact treatment will depend on the cause and the nature of the wound. The vast majority of lacerations simply require closure with glue, adhesive skin closures or sutures. Other common minor injury treatments include:

Avulsion of nail

- Eliminate other underlying damage, control bleeding.
- Remove nail or partial avulsion of nail only when the nail is very loose, easily removable and restoration of normal alignment is not possible (Moulton and Yates 1999).
- Whenever possible replant the nail back into the nail bed and secure with sutures or adhesive strips (Keltie 1996). Dress and leave in place for 7 days.
- Review every 2–3 days.

Pre-tibial lacerations

Most pre-tibial lacerations should not be sutured. Use adhesive skin strips (Moulton and Yates 1999). However the young person with thicker pre-tibial flaps are better treated by suturing (Keltie 1997).

Burns and scalds

- Erythema does not require dressing but analgesia should be advised.
- Dressings are only required if the wound is partial thickness.
- De-roofing of blisters is controversial and while some authors recommend de-roofing others suggest small blisters should be left intact and large blisters punctured but the skin left as a dressing.
- Facial – dress with liquid paraffin for first 24–48 h provided inhalation injury has been excluded.

- Body and limbs – dress with a non-adherent dressing for first 36–48 h and review (Moulton and Yates 1999).
- Hand burns – flamazine is applied and a loose fitting glove or bag is taped around the wrist (Moulton and Yates 1999).

BITES – HUMAN AND ANIMAL

- Most bites should be left open (Howarth and Evans 1994). Due to the excellent blood supply and need for cosmetic appearance facial wounds can be sutured/adhesive strips (Moulton and Yates 1999).
- Insect bites should be treated with Flucloxacillin and Penicillin.
- All human, dog and cat bites causing a breach of the skin require antibiotic therapy such as erythromycin or co-amoxiclav (Moulton and Yates 1999).
- Review ALL bites after 24 h.
- Remember tetanus prophylaxis.

Fish hooks

Fish hooks can often become embedded into the skin (normally the finger)
- Push the barb through the skin (local anaesthetic may be required)
- Cut the barb using wire cutters
- Withdraw the cut hook
- Clean and dress the wound.

MINOR ILLNESSES

The number of minor illnesses that present at a walk in centre or GP surgery is beyond the remit of this book, however a number of common themes can be identified and general assessment and treatment highlighted.

SKIN CONDITIONS/RASHES

The history and general examination of the patient's overall physical condition is essential when assessing any skin condition. Often a skin condition/rash is one sign of a systemic disorder.

Assessment and treatment
- Painful vesicles turning to pustules/crusting and following a sensory nerve suggests shingles – treatment is with one of the antiviral agents.
- Erythematous papules and vesicles that weep, ooze and encrust commonly on the scalp and flexor surfaces of joints is suggestive of eczema – topical steroids are the most common forms of treatment.
- Local rash with some swelling and urticaria is common in contact dermatitis – often removal of the contact agent and a simple emollient is sufficient.
- Rashes that cover large areas of the body can be due to a range of infections from rubella to meningitis – treatment/referral will depend on the type of rash and local protocols.
- Warts/growths on the skin are often benign but could be basal cell or squamous cell carcinoma. Basal cell carcinoma tends to have a nodular pigmented appearance while squamous cell carcinoma is red, scaly and has a sharp demarcated border.

EAR/NOSE/THROAT AND RESPIRATORY RELATED CONDITIONS

Assessment and treatment
- *Colds and Flu* are traditionally seen in the winter and locally there are normally a large number of people affected. Coughing, sneezing, joint aches; high temperature and weakness are all common symptoms. Colds are normally self-limiting while flu can continue for several weeks – treatment is symptomatic.
- *Sinusitis* causes congestion and heaviness in the face. The sinuses can become painful especially on palpation. Postnasal drip may also cause distress especially at night – treatment includes decongestant sprays and if the sinuses are infected antibiotics.
- *Earache* can be due to a number of disorders.
- *Otitis externa* – red swollen tissue in the external canal that may obscure the tympanic membrane – treatment antibiotics/analgesia

- *Otitis* media – bacterial is often seen as a red, thickened and bulging tympanic membrane – treatment antibiotics/analgesia.
- *Wax* is seen in the external canal – treatment includes softening the wax and then ear syringing.
- *Throat infections* can range from simple viral infections to tonsillitis. Simple redness of the oropharynx suggests a simple pharyngitis. Hoarseness may suggest laryngitis. Swollen, red tonsils with or without exudate can indicate infection – treatment is symptomatic and may also include antibiotics.
- *Difficulty with breathing* can be due to simple cold/nasal congestion through to a major respiratory condition. It is essential that any patient complaining of difficulty with breathing be fully assessed including percussion and auscultation.

HEADACHES

A headache is a symptom of an underlying disorder rather than a disease in itself (Walsh 1999).

While the headache may reflect a serious neurological disorder it is more commonly due to eyestrain, tension, migraine or a nasal/sinus problem.

Assessment must include a full neurological examination and visual acuity. The description and history will often help with the diagnosis.

Eyestrain	often dull aching around the eyes, poor visual acuity, can be worse at twilight/at night
Tension	often related to neck muscle spasm, position, activity, anxiety
Migraine	localized pain, nausea, vomiting, visual disturbances

Treatment is symptomatic.

OTHER COMMON COMPLAINTS THAT MAY OR MAY NOT BE OF A MINOR NATURE

Abdominal pain and urinary disorders can often be short-term problems caused by a 24-h viral infection or due to a bacterial infection that is treated with a course of antibiotics. The range of viral and bacterial infections that affect the gastro-intestinal tract can debilitate an individual not only with the recognized symptoms of diarrhoea and vomiting but also systemically.

What appears to be a minor illness such as "heartburn" could be a symptom of an ulcer. What appears to be a simple bout of "indigestion" could be a myocardial infarction. The key to determining the minor from the major has to be found in the history, the examination and the result of simple treatments.

CONCLUSION

This chapter has covered a number of minor injuries/illness that are commonly seen in the emergency care setting. It is essential that an in depth assessment is always undertaken to ensure that what may appear to be a minor injury is such and not a major problem waiting to happen.

References

British National Formulary (1999) BMA and Royal Pharmaceutical Society.

Chong N, Murray P (1993) Pen torch test in patients with unilateral red eye. *Br J Genl Prac* 43(371): 259.

Dale J, Dolan B (1996) Do patients use minor injuries units appropriately? *J Public Health Med* 18(2): 152–156.

Dawson D, Sanders K (2000) In: Dolan B, Holt L, eds. *Accident and emergency theory into practice*. London: Bailliere Tindall.

Driscoll P et al (1993) *Trauma resuscitation the team approach*. London: Macmillan Press.

Heaney D (1997) Evaluation of a nurse-led minor injuries unit. *Nurs Stand* 12(4): 35–38.

Hoffman JR, Mower WR, Wolfson AB et al (2000) Validity of clinical criteria to rule out injury to the cervical spine in patients with blunt trauma. *New Engl J Med* 343: 94–99.

Howarth P, Evans R (1994) *Key topics in accident and emergency medicine*. Oxford: Bios Scientific Publishers.

Jones G (1993) Minor injury care in the community. *Nurs Stand* 7(22): 35–36.

Keltie D (1996) The A–Z of hand injuries. *3M A&E Focus*. Issues 2/3/4.

Keltie D (1997) Managing pre-tibial lacerations – a different approach in young and old? *3M A&E Focus*. Issue 5 (Spring).

McElvanney A, Fielder A (1993) Intraocular foreign body missed by radiography. *Br Med J* 306(6884): 1060–1061.

Moulton C, Yates D (1999) *Lecture notes on emergency medicine*. Oxford: Blackwell Science.

Paxton F (1997) Minor injuries units: evaluating patients' perceptions. *Nurs Stand* 12(5): 45–47.

Vinson DR (2001) NEXUS cervical spine criteria. *Ann Emergen Med* 37(2): 237–238.

Walsh M (1999) In: Walsh M, Crumbie A, Reveley S, eds. *Nurse practitioners clinical skills and professional issues*. Oxford: Butterworth Heinemann.

Wardrope J, English B (1998) *Musculo-skeletal problems in emergency medicine*. Oxford: Oxford University Press.

Watts BL, Armstrong B (2001) A randomised controlled trial to determine the effectiveness of double Tubigrip in grade 1 and 2 (mild to moderate) ankle sprains. *Emergen Med J* 18: 46–50.

Westaby S (1985) *Wound care*. London: William Heinemann.

Wilderness Medical Associates (2000) Presentation by Handlan M at *Emergency Nurses Association Conference* USA 2000.

Gary Jones

9 | Major disasters and major incidents

Mike Hayward

"We all live in a world of our own, surrounded by a protective cocoon that isolates us from most of the major problems that other people have. If you work in a hospital, you acknowledge that major disasters are going to occur, but it is unlikely that they will affect your hospital – you hope these things happen to others."   Wallace (1994)

INTRODUCTION

Disaster has many faces: the Bradford football stadium fire, the Ladbroke Grove train crash, the sinking of the Herald of Free Enterprise off Zeebruge, the chemical leak at Bhopal in India, the radiation leak at Chernobyl, the Omagh bombing. The list appears endless. The key to dealing effectively with disasters or major incidents is through preparedness and good management.

The tragic terrorist attacks in the USA on September 11th 2001, served to focus worldwide attention on the potential and widespread methods of attack that fanatical terrorists can, and will employ (The Times 2001). More worryingly, the subsequent anthrax incidents, and associated fatalities, gave a wake up call to disaster planners across the world (BBC 2001). These terrorist attacks in the United States have required a revision of the basic assumptions underlying the civil contingency planning arrangements, at all levels within the UK. This has resulted in a renewed interest in health service disaster planning and has helped refocus attention on an often-ignored area of emergency care.

Although rare events, it is important that all Emergency Departments have contingency plans to deal with major incidents or major disasters that occur within their geographical area (Carley and Mackway-Jones 1996; NHSE 1998). Current NHS guidance for English NHS Trusts and Health Authorities is laid down in the handbook, *Planning for major incidents* (NHSE 1998). This guidance requires all NHS Trusts to have a major incident plan that considers all foreseeable causes of a major incident, and all aspects of the hospitals response. Guidance for Northern Ireland can be found in a Public Safety Unit Circular PSU1/2000 (DHSS 2000), for Scotland in the *Manual of guidance: responding to emergencies* (NHS in Scotland 1998) and for Wales in the document, *Planning for major incidents: the NHS guidance* (NHS Service Directorate for the National Assembly for Wales 1999). A major disaster/incident plan is intended to provide optimum treatment of the victims of a major accident when there are too many patients to be dealt with by the routine emergency services (Bliss 1984). The global organization of disaster planning in the NHS is summarized in Figure 9.1 (p. 154).

Although rare, major incidents can, and do happen. It is therefore important that Emergency Departments are ready to efficiently and effectively deal with them if they do. Disaster preparedness is an important training issue for emergency nurses, particularly since various papers have highlighted the poor standard of preparation for major incidents in the UK (Cooke 1992; Nancekievill 1992; Carley and Mackway-Jones 1996). Few health care professionals will experience more than one major incident, and most will never be involved in any throughout their whole careers (Eaton 1999). Unfortunately therefore, many nurses adopt the attitude that it will never happen in their department. Indeed, that is probably what a majority of emergency nurses on duty in any of the hospitals in Manchester on 15th June 1996 thought, until the largest bomb ever detonated on mainland Britain exploded. By the end of their shifts, the nurses working in the six Emergency Departments would have

Major disasters and major incidents

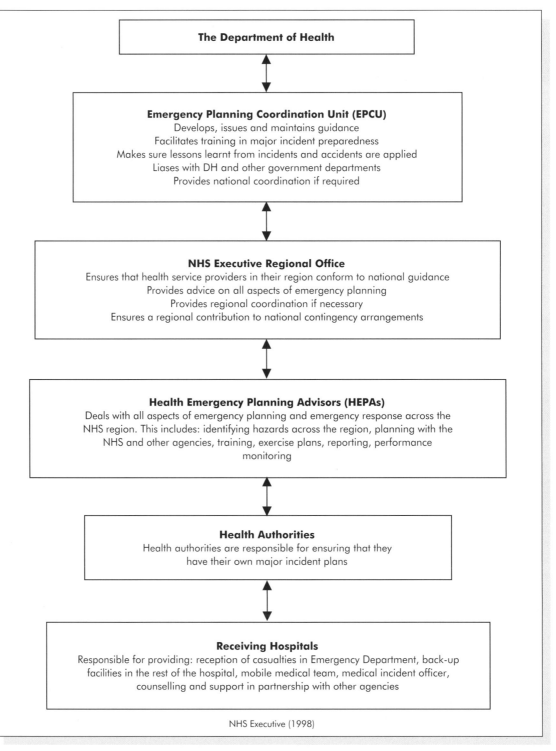

The Department of Health

Emergency Planning Coordination Unit (EPCU)
Develops, issues and maintains guidance
Facilitates training in major incident preparedness
Makes sure lessons learnt from incidents and accidents are applied
Liases with DH and other government departments
Provides national coordination if required

NHS Executive Regional Office
Ensures that health service providers in their region conform to national guidance
Provides advice on all aspects of emergency planning
Provides regional coordination if necessary
Ensures a regional contribution to national contingency arrangements

Health Emergency Planning Advisors (HEPAs)
Deals with all aspects of emergency planning and emergency response across the
NHS region. This includes: identifying hazards across the region, planning with the
NHS and other agencies, training, exercise plans, reporting, performance
monitoring

Health Authorities
Health authorities are responsible for ensuring that they
have their own major incident plans

Receiving Hospitals
Responsible for providing: reception of casualties in Emergency Department, back-up
facilities in the rest of the hospital, mobile medical team, medical incident officer,
counselling and support in partnership with other agencies

NHS Executive (1998)

Figure 9.1 The organization of disaster planning in the NHS

treated over 200 casualties between them (Carley and Mackway-Jones 1997).

DISASTER OR MAJOR INCIDENT?

Before addressing the role of the nurse in the major incident/disaster situation it is necessary to examine the definitions and differences between the terms disaster and major incident. With regard to incidents such as the 1989 Kegworth plane crash and the 1989 Hillsborough stadium crush, it has been suggested by the Advanced Life Support Group (ALSG) (1995), that the terms major disaster and major incident are often used loosely and interchangeably. Therefore, a greater exploration of the two concepts is needed in order to minimize confusion of terminology.

The very definition of disaster is problematic, as there is much debate and controversy over the true meaning of disaster. The word appears to be applicable to everything from an event like an earthquake to occasions when two ladies turn up for a party wearing the same dress (Rutherford and de Boer 1983). Tierney (1989, pp. 11–12) asserts that, members of the general public, researchers and practitioners use the word disaster in several different ways.

The New Shorter Oxford English Dictionary (1993) defines disaster as, "sudden or great misfortune; an event of ruinous or distressing nature, a calamity" (p. 683). The *Readers Digest Universal Dictionary* (1991) adds the element of destruction to the definition by suggesting that disaster is, "an occurrence inflicting widespread destruction and distress; a grave misfortune" (p. 442). Whereas the League of Red Cross and Red Crescent Societies (1985) (cited in The World Health Organisation 1999) provides a more holistic and nursing focused definition in their assertion that, "a disaster is a catastrophic situation in which the day-to-day patterns of life are disrupted and people are plunged into helplessness and suffering and, as a result, need protection, water, food, clothing, shelter, medical and social care, and other necessities of life" (p. 2).

The ALSG (1995) recommend that the term "disaster" be reserved for events that produce a wider disturbance in the community, other than the need for special arrangements by the emergency services – they suggest for example, an earthquake or flood. This recommendation appears both prescriptive and

very limiting, failing to consider the long-term psychiatric effects on survivors, families and relief workers, not to mention the effects on the community as a whole, following such traumatic incidents as the 1985 Bradford stadium fire or the 1989 Hillsborough stadium crush. What for some was a serious major incident, may well have become an ongoing psychological disaster for others. The term "major incident" applied to most things other than large natural disasters conjures up a limiting sense of *"short-termism"*; the danger of which is failure to encapsulate the wider reaching and longer-term effects of the incident (Davis and Stewart 2000). Health service personnel, particularly psychiatric and community nurses, are involved in incidents such as Hillsborough for many months, and sometimes years after the event (Hinks 1993).

The term "disaster" is not routinely used in the UK; the Department of Health prefers to use the term "major incident" (Ryan and Gavalas 1998). A major incident in the health service has been defined as, "an event that owing to the number and severity of live casualties requires special arrangements by the health service" (NHSME 1990). This can encompass incidents such as the 1996 *E. coli* infection outbreak in Lanarkshire or the 1996 boiler room flood at University College Hospital, London, where 202 patients had to be transferred to other hospitals and the Emergency Department closed to emergencies (NHSE 1998). It is also important to remember that a major incident for one emergency service may not apply to all other emergency services (NHSE 1998; ALSG 1995). The classic major incident, which stretched all the emergency services, was the Kegworth air crash in 1989. A plane carrying 126 people crashed on the M1 motorway in England, killing 47 of the occupants and injuring 79. The ambulance service had to provide 181 ambulance personnel, 14 officers and 75 vehicles. The three receiving hospitals had to deal with 82 casualties, who between them had sustained 191 fractures, as well as many other serious injuries (NHSE 1998).

INCIDENCE AND TYPES OF DISASTERS

The Emergency Events Database (EM-DAT) at the Centre for Research on the Epidemiology of Disasters (CRED), University of Louvain, Brussels shows that

Table 9.1
Notable British major incidents (adapted from Carley et al 1998)

Year	Incident	Dead at scene	Seen and discharged from Emergency Department	Total injured and dead
1915	Train crash at Quintinshill	227		427
1968	Ronan point tower block crash	4	14	21
1973	Fire at Summerland complex, IOM	48	86	150
1974	Chemical explosion, Flixborough	28	>200	>250
1974	Tavern in the Town pub bombing, Birmingham	11	56	100
1975	Moorgate tube crash	43	56	115
1983	Harrods bomb, London	5		95
1985	Manchester air crash	52	60	137
1985	Bradford football stadium fire	52	181	308
1987	Kings Cross underground fire	31		91
1987	Multiple rta, M4 motorway	4		78
1988	Clapham train crash	35		123
1989	Air crash, Kegworth	47	5	126
1989	Crowd crush, Hillsborough stadium	81	69	240
1989	Marchioness pleasure boat sinking, London	51		131
1991	Cannon Street station, train crash	2	507	542
1999	Ladbroke Grove train crash	31		431
2000	Hatfield train crash	4		74
2001	Selby, train crash	10		86

- Transport
  - Rail
  - Road
  - Maritime
  - Aviation
- Industrial
  - Chemical
  - Mining
  - Construction
  - Nuclear
- War and terrorist incidents
- Civil disorder/riots
- Crowd accidents

Figure 9.2 Human-initiated disasters

Earthquake
Volcanic eruptions
Tornado
Floods
Drought
Tsunami
Famine
Pestilence
Heat wave
Natural fire
Famine

Figure 9.3 Natural disasters

in 1999 there were 623 reported disasters worldwide, resulting in approximately 80,404 deaths, with a staggering 212,544,647 people affected by those disasters (cited in: International Federation of Red Cross and Red Crescent Societies 2000). Fortunately, due to both its geographical position and relative economic prosperity, the UK suffers relatively few disasters. However, it has been suggested that there are on average three or four major incidents per year occurring in the UK (Table 9.1) (Carley et al 1998).

Disasters can be broadly categorized as natural or human initiated (see Figures 9.2 and 9.3). In the UK, most disasters are human initiated because, as well as occupying a temperate geographic position, high level societies such as the UK, usually take on preventative measures and reduce secondary effects with sound infrastructure and adequate financing (Lumley 1998). However, it is dangerous to become complacent in the UK and ignore the potential threat of natural disasters. A historical examination of extreme

Avalanche: Eight killed when a cornice of frozen snow broke away and fell 60 m onto houses in Lewes, East Sussex, 27 December 1836.
Flood: 2000 died around the Severn Estuary, 20 January 1606.
Smog: 3500–4000 died, mostly children and the elderly, from bronchitis caused by smog in London, 4–9 December 1952.
Storm: Approximately 8000 killed by "The Channel Storm" of 26 November 1703.
Whirlwind: 74 killed when train plunged into sea from Tay Bridge (Tayside), after bridge collapsed under impact of two or three waterspouts, 28 December 1879.

Figure 9.4 UK catastrophes caused by extreme weather (Torro.co.uk, undated)

British weather phenomena graphically illustrates this (see Figure 9.4). Also, while the UK is nowhere near in the same league as California, Taiwan or Japan in terms of major earthquake activity, it nevertheless has a moderate rate of seismic activity; sufficiently high to pose a potential hazard to sensitive installations such as, nuclear power stations, dams and chemical plants (Geologyshop.com, undated).

DECLARING A MAJOR INCIDENT

"A major incident is a high profile event which places the emergency services in the spotlight of public attention at a time of great strain"   (New 1992).

Any of the emergency services may declare a major incident, or any NHS hospital that feels that the NHS definition of a major incident has been met, can also declare a major incident (Whitfield and Kilner 2000). The ALSG (1995) raise the issue of reluctance to declare a major incident citing, professional pride, fear of criticism for calling a major incident unnecessarily or ignorance, as the major reasons. This behaviour is wholly unacceptable and, if in any doubt, a major incident should always be declared. It is much easier to stand staff and resources down, than to try and muster staff and resources well into a developing major incident or disaster when minutes could mean the difference between life and death.

Within the NHS, it is usually the ambulance service that notifies a designated receiving hospital's switchboard of a major incident (NHSE 1998; Hodgetts

Bradford stadium fire 1985
Manchester airport fire 1985
Hungerford massacre 1987
Canary Wharf 1996

Figure 9.5 Unannounced major incidents

"Major incident – stand by"
This alerts a hospital that a major incident is possibly imminent. Notify key staff only.

"Major incident declared – activate plan"
The incident has occurred. A full response is required.

"Major incident – cancelled"
There is no longer the threat of a major incident and rescinds either of the first two messages at any time.

"Major incident – casualty evacuation complete"
All receiving hospitals are alerted as soon as all casualties have been removed from the site; the ambulance incident officer will make it clear if any casualties are still en route.

Figure 9.6 Standardized major incident messages (ALSG, 1995; NHSE 1998; Hodgetts and Miles 2000)

and Miles 2000). Although the ambulance service are the most common declarers of NHS major incidents, Emergency Department staff must also be mindful that they may get no official notification of an incident occurring (Walsh 1990). This can happen when a disaster takes place in the local vicinity of a hospital such as the 1987 King Cross underground fire and the 1989 Hillsborough stadium crush (NHSE 1998). Figure 9.5 shows other examples of major incidents that were self-declared by the hospital or in which there were problems with communication.

If a major incident is declared by anyone other than the ambulance service, the ambulance service must be notified immediately (NHSE 1998). Failure of communication from the scene of major incidents, and also between the emergency services, has been regularly cited as an important weakness in the response to actual major incidents (Fennell 1988; Hidden 1989; Marriott 1991; Lloyd 1991). Due to this, the notifying messages that hospitals receive from the other emergency services have been standardized and are the only ones that should ever be used with regard to major incident notification; these are shown in Figure 9.6.

MOBILE MEDICAL TEAMS

Current NHS guidance, *Planning for major incidents* (NHSE 1998), requires nominated acute hospitals to provide a trained and equipped mobile medical team (MMT) to attend the site of a major incident if requested. Surprisingly, the concept of the mobile medical team in the UK has been around since at least 1954 when the Ministry of Health issued formal guidance on 'Medical Arrangements for Dealing with Major Accidents' (Hines 1997). The role of the MMT is confined to rapid assessment, life-saving procedures and organizing rapid removal to hospital for those casualties who will benefit most from such prioritization (Salt 1989). Deployment of a medical and nursing team must clearly be perceived to benefit patient care at the site of the incident, otherwise the team should remain at the hospital where they can be more effectively utilized (Kilner 2000).

The ambulance service is responsible for requesting the despatch of an MMT to the scene of a major incident. It is good practice for the ambulance service to try to avoid requesting an MMT from the main receiving hospital so as not to deplete existing resources (ALSG 1995). However, in very rural locations, the local district general hospital may have to be the receiving hospital and also send an MMT (Eaton 1999).

Traditionally, the MMT is made up of Emergency Department personnel usually supported by an anaesthetist. An MMT is made up of four members; an experienced doctor (Registrar or above) to act as team leader, an anaesthetist, a senior emergency nurse and a second experienced nurse (Eaton 1999).

The ALSG (1995) reinforce the fact that it is no longer acceptable to approach the scene of a major incident as enthusiastic amateurs. If the team is inexperienced, unskilled, ill-equipped, or undisciplined then it can become a burden rather than an asset (ALSG 1995). Unfortunately, research by Moakes and Kilner (2001) highlighted that many emergency nurses had little knowledge of what their role would be as part of an MMT, and concluded that they appeared inadequately prepared.

Therefore, where possible, the team leader should have attended a major incident medical management course (MIMMS), both the doctors should have attended a pre-hospital care course and all members of the team should be trained in their appropriate

advanced life support course whether it be Advanced Trauma Life Support (ATLS), Pre-Hospital Trauma Life Support (PHTLS) or the Trauma Nurse Care Course (TNCC) (Hodgetts and Miles 2000).

When assembling an MMT, careful consideration must be given to the issue of getting the right nurses to the scene without reducing the effectiveness of the Emergency Department or hospital generally (Salt 1989).

Various authors (Fletcher 1986; Kilner 1996; McGregor et al 1997) have questioned the safety of MMTs. Members of an MMT called on to work at the scene of a major incident are required to operate in an unfamiliar, hostile and inherently dangerous environment (Kilner 1996; Graham and Hearns 1999). The scene of a disaster is alien to most nurses, as the hospital setting is a moderately quiet, controlled and relatively safe environment. Most major incident scenes pose a serious threat to rescuers, whether it is from flammable fluids such as petrol, sharp fragments from damaged vehicles or the risk of infection from body fluids (Norton 1998). It is therefore essential that all members of an MMT are adequately and safely attired when despatched to an incident scene (see Figure 9.7).

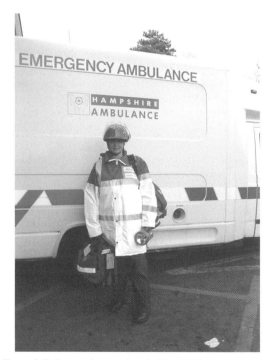

Figure 9.7 Personal protective clothing MMT

Warm underclothing
Fire retardant boiler suit
High visibility waterproof jacket marked "NURSE" front
and back
High visibility waistcoat marked "NURSE" front and
back (warm weather)
Green helmet with visor marked "NURSE"
Miners headlight
Thick gloves (protection against sharp metal, etc.)
Surgical gloves
Oil and acid-resistant steel toe capped boots
(preferably leather)
Ear defenders

Figure 9.8 Personal protective clothing for nurses

The Health and Safety at Work Act (HSE 1974) places legal responsibilities upon employers to ensure, so far as is reasonably practicable, the health, safety and welfare at work of all employees. Current guidance states that the Ambulance Safety Officer or the Medical Incident Officer (MIO) should refuse inappropriately dressed staff access to the major incident scene (ALSG 1995). Figure 9.8 gives details of minimum standards of safety dress for nurse members of an MMT.

THE SCENE OF A MAJOR INCIDENT

It is important for all emergency nurses who are likely to be part of an MMT to have an understanding of command and control at a major incident scene. Years of practice and lessons learnt from past mistakes, have lead to a standardized management approach to the command of major incidents. In order to maximize efficiency and maintain control over a potentially chaotic situation there is necessarily a hierarchical, and military like, command structure. At a major incident scene there will be an inner cordon, where the rescue operation is actually taking place, and an outer cordon, which surrounds the whole of the incident including the command vehicles. There are three tiers of command, known as bronze, silver and gold. Bronze control is "operational" and is the area directly around the major incident site itself, or in layman's terms, the "coal face". Silver control is "tactical" and is where all emergency services set up their emergency control vehicles. Each emergency service will appoint a senior officer as an incident officer who is

normally located within silver control. Silver incident officers may also move inside the bronze areas. Gold control is "strategic" and is remote from the scene, where chief officers monitor and control the wider picture (ALSG 1995; Hodgetts and Miles 2000).

The doctor in command at the scene is known as the MIO (Medical Incident Officer) and is usually located around the incident control point at silver level. The MIO has no direct contact with casualties in order to allow the MIO to concentrate solely on control, support and logistics. The MIO wears a green and white chequered tabard labelled "MEDICAL INCIDENT OFFICER". All MMT members must report to the MIO on arrival at the scene. The overall control of the major incident scene is the responsibility of the Police Service. However, the overall safety of the scene is the responsibility of the Fire and Rescue Service and therefore, they are often in charge at Bronze (operational) level. All nursing staff are arriving at the scene of a major incident work under the orders of the MIO or the Forward MIO.

MAJOR INCIDENT TRIAGE

Any nurse deployed to the scene of a major incident needs to have an awareness and understanding of disaster triage. Most emergency nurses are used to conventional triage and the concepts behind it. A majority of Emergency Departments use a standard five-point triage scale (Crouch and Marrow 1996) or approaches such as the Manchester Triage system (Mackway-Jones 1996). Major disaster triage utilizes the philosophy of doing, "the most for the most" and can appear brutal and callous to the uninitiated. Time and resources cannot be tied up attending to casualties who are identified as likely to die, as this will distract resources from those who are likely to live (Hodgetts and Miles 2000). Therefore, it is essential that in a mass casualty situation, patients with probable non-survivable injuries such as 80% burns or bilateral high traumatic amputation of legs, be left to one side in order that other patients with a greater chance of survival are transported to hospital first (Walsh 1990). Disaster triage is based on military battlefield triage and has five categories:

Red **Priority 1 (Immediate)**
– Casualties   requiring   immediate   life-saving
procedures.

Major disasters and major incidents

	Trauma score							Expected (untreated) % survival
Red	1–10	Priority 1	P1	Critical	Immediate	T1	10
Yellow	11	Priority 2	P2	Serious	Urgent	T2	30
Green	12	Priority 3	P3	Minor	Delayed	T3	60
Blue	0				Expectant	T4	None
White				Dead	Deceased	T0	

Figure 9.9 Triage categories (adapted from Eaton (1999))

Yellow Priority 2 (Urgent)
– Casualties requiring intervention within 4–6 h.

Green Priority 3 (Delayed)
– "Walking wounded" who do not require urgent treatment.

Blue Priority 4 (Expectant)
– Only used in major mass casualty situations. Casualties whose injuries are so severe that they cannot survive in the circumstances.

White Dead

A more detailed understanding of the battlefield triage categories can be seen in Figure 9.9. It must be remembered that triage is a dynamic process and reassessment must be carried out as practicable. The initial triage decision is usually made on the actual scene of the major incident and is known as the triage sieve. Paramedics or doctors usually carry this out. Subsequent decisions are carried out in the casualty clearing station by a doctor and are known as the triage sort (ALSG 1995). Once triaged, patients should have a cruciform triage label showing their category firmly attached to their person (see Figure 9.10).

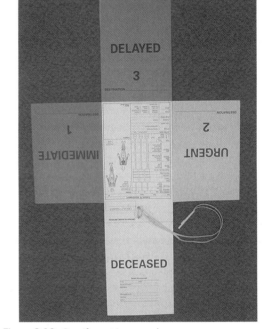

Figure 9.10 Cruciform triage card

THE EMERGENCY DEPARTMENT HOSPITAL RESPONSE

As soon as the "major incident declared" message is received, or initiated by a hospital itself, the hospital major incident plan is brought into action. Hospital major incident plans are necessarily large and complex documents, as they have to legislate for the rapid transformation of a routine hospital service into a temporary widespread emergency service, with as little disruption and compromise to patient safety as possible. A hospital major incident control room will be set up in the pre-designated location. This is manned by senior hospital staff including, a senior clinician, a senior manager and a senior nurse, and acts as the hospital's nerve centre during the major incident.

All hospital major incident plans will be different, due to the varying sizes of, and services offered by, different UK district general hospitals. Readers are therefore advised to study their own hospitals' major incident plan, for a greater understanding of the required actions from various staff and departments, during an activated major incident.

Patients already in the Emergency Department awaiting treatment for minor injuries when a major incident is declared, should be given any appropriate first aid if needed and then advised to go home, attend another out of area Emergency Department or see their GP as appropriate. More seriously injured, unstable or ill patients should be rapidly stabilized and transferred to a ward (Walsh 1990; Whitfield and Kilner 2000).

It should be remembered that even though a major incident has happened, this does not stop other accidents or injuries from occurring locally and critically ill patients can, and do, still arrive at the Emergency Department. This is graphically illustrated by Clifton (1994, p. 108) who, whilst writing about the Kegworth air crash, noted that:

"just because there had been an air crash on the M1 didn't stop people fighting in pubs, crashing their cars on the A46, or having a coronary".

To effectively manage an Emergency Department during a major incident it is important to ensure that all casualties arrive through one entrance (NHSE 1998). In most Emergency Departments this will be the ambulance bay entrance, and all other entrances into the department should be closed. The process of prioritization of casualties should have begun at the scene, but it must be repeated and performed accurately if the most seriously injured are to have access to scarce critical care facilities (Ryan and Gavalas 1998). Therefore, a triage receiving station should be set up at this entrance to the Emergency Department and the senior Emergency Department doctor present becomes the Chief Triage Officer assisted by an experienced triage nurse. The Chief Triage Officer is responsible for re-triaging all patients as they arrive and sending them to the appropriate treatment area of the Emergency Department (Hodgetts and Miles 2000).

On receipt of a major incident declared message, a designated person will start to call in off duty staff as dictated by the size and scale of the incident involved. The senior clinical emergency nurse present will take overall control of the department. There is no place for non-clinical managers attempting to co-ordinate and manage a clinical area during a major incident, they should be supplying the Emergency Department with back up facilities such as extra equipment, trolleys and pairs of hands (Walsh 1990).

Action cards containing clear and concise written instructions for each individuals' role in a major incident should be easily located within the department (Sleet 1989). The senior nurse will ensure that all staff, from consultants to receptionists, are provided with the necessary action card, detailing their exact role during the major incident (see Figure 9.11). Emergency Department staff that have been called in, must report to the nurse in charge of the department so that they can be allocated to an appropriate area. It is imperative to the success of the major incident plan that they remain in that post unless redeployed by the nurse in charge. Where possible, all Emergency Department staff should wear an identification tabard, displaying their title, in order to assist unfamiliar members of hospital staff to identify key equipment and supplies (Hodgetts and Miles 2000; Whitfield and Kilner 2000).

Regular Emergency Department staff will be divided into treatment teams. A treatment team should comprise of two doctors and two nurses, with at least one of the nurses being an emergency nurse. Each Priority 1, or immediate need, casualty will require a dedicated treatment team until stabilized and transferred. However, it should be possible to care for two, or three, Priority 2, or urgent need, casualties with one treatment team depending on the types of injury involved (Whitfield and Kilner 2000).

Major incidents attract large numbers of non-hospital staff to the receiving hospitals such as non-medical volunteers, members of the press, freelance photographers, "do-gooders", untrained impostors and voyeurs. In order to facilitate order and control, it is important to limit access to the hospital and to ensure that a security cordon is established around the Emergency Department. Therefore, all staff called in will have to be in possession of their hospital ID card or access may well be refused by the police or hospital security. Occasionally, the involvement of radioactivity or chemical and/or biological agents may well complicate major incidents. It is therefore important that emergency nurses have an understanding of these rare, but potentially hazardous occurrences.

INCIDENTS INVOLVING RADIATION

Major incidents involving radiation are rare anywhere in the world. However, when they do occur they can be catastrophic and affect large numbers of people. In 1986, a nuclear reactor explosion in Chernobyl, USSR killed at least 32 people and contaminated 116,000 others (Clarke 1987). Ricks and

---

MAJOR INCIDENT ACTION CARD   EMERGENCY DEPARTMENT

NURSE-IN-CHARGE OF EMERGENCY DEPARTMENT BED AREA (MAJOR AREA 2)

1 With Emergency Department Consultant clear the Observation Ward of patients and prepare to receive casualties.
2 Deploy staff throughout the Emergency Department bed area, taking into account patient dependency.
3 Confer regularly with Major Incident Control Centre, Emergency Department regarding:
   a. Staffing requirements
   b. Need for other equipment and supplies
   c. Workload and nature of injuries
   d. Arrangements for meal and rest periods

Major Incident Control Centre Numbers – 6010, 6020, 6023

NOTE: Recognition of Staff and Volunteers

Identifying tabards or armbands will be worn as follows:

Tabards	Red	–	Medical
	Blue	–	Nursing
	Green	–	Administrative and Clerical
Armbands	Yellow	–	Volunteers

ISSUE 4. AUGUST 2001   *REMEMBER YOUR SECURITY CARD*   8 OF 28

RECORD YOUR ACTIONS   **RECORD YOUR ACTIONS**   **RECORD YOUR ACTIONS**

Portsmouth Hospitals NHS Trust

Figure 9.11 Example of major incident action card

Fry (1990) identified 15 separate radiation accidents involving fatalities between the years 1981 and 1993, which highlights the need for preparedness.

Emergency Eepartments located close to nuclear power stations or fixed nuclear sites such as Dungeness, Sizewell A or Sellafield, should be well practised and trained in dealing with potential nuclear accidents (NHSE 1998). However, it is probably a fair assumption to make that many emergency nurses, working in other departments, know little about radiation injuries or contaminated casualties.

It is therefore important for emergency nurses to be aware that nuclear material is transported every day by road, rail, sea and air, which gives the potential for a nuclear accident anywhere at any time (Eaton 1999). In fact, it is estimated that some 38 million packages of radioactive material are shipped worldwide per year (British Energy undated). More worryingly, Smith (1995) highlights the trade in smuggled plutonium, a practice that in itself poses serious potential health risks, but also raises the concern of a nuclear weapon being made and detonated by a terrorist

Accident at a nuclear power station
Spillage of medical isotopes in transit
Accident involving nuclear waste or fissile in transit
Accident involving nuclear warheads in transit or at a
   military establishment
Nuclear bomb – war or terrorism

Figure 9.12 Potential types of radioactive incident

group. Figure 9.12 shows the types of incident that could potentially result in radioactive contaminated casualties.

UNDERSTANDING RADIATION

Hospitals prepared to accept radiation casualties and to assist with decontamination of personnel should be designated by all health authorities (NHSE 1998). Hospitals not equipped to deal with incidents involving radioactivity can request specialist monitoring, assessment and decontamination skills via the police through the National Arrangements for Incidents involving Radiation (NAIR) Scheme. Fong and Schrader (1996) highlight the medical profession's relative ignorance in terms of dealing with radiation accidents, believing that most health care professionals find it difficult to, "understand the comparison of radiation exposures gained from a chest radiograph, a transatlantic flight, or the Three Mile Island accident". To confidently and competently manage casualties of radiation accidents it is therefore important for nurses to have a basic understanding of radioactivity.

Radiation is the transfer of energy through space; it is all around us, for example in light and heat, most of which causes us little harm (Walsh 1989; Fong and Schrader 1996). Radiation reaches earth from outer space, the earth itself is radioactive and naturally occurring radionuclides are present in the air we breathe, in the food we eat and in our own bodies (Fry 1987). However, certain types of radiation, such as ionizing radiation, are dangerous as it can disrupt the atomic structure of material it encounters (Walsh 1989). Ionizing radiation is radiation that can produce charged ions in any material it strikes. Where ionization occurs in molecules that are present in living cells, biological damage may result. Ionizing radiation may be generated from a variety of sources, which may be particle emitting or electromagnetic (Wythe 1999). Steedman (1994) identifies that biological damage can be caused by five types of ionizing radiation which are illustrated in Figure 9.13.

Radiation casualties can either be irradiated or contaminated. The two different terms need to be fully understood by emergency nurses if safe and effective treatment is to be administered. A person who has been irradiated poses no threat to others as they have been exposed to radiation but it has passed through them and they contain no radioactive material on their person. These casualties may be treated in a normal way in the Emergency Department, but will need careful in-hospital monitoring depending what aspect of radiation sickness develops (Walsh 1990). However, a person who has been contaminated has radioactive material on their clothes, on their skin, or inside them if it has ingested or inhaled (Walsh 1989). In other words a contaminated casualty is still emitting radiation and is a danger to others. Precautions will therefore be required to minimize the spread of contamination to attendants, vehicles, and the treatment facilities (Steedman 1994). If there

---

Alpha particles: Can only travel a few centimetres in air. Cannot penetrate through the epidermal layer of the skin. Damage can follow ingestion, inhalation or absorption of alpha emitting substances through an open wound. Therefore alpha particles constitute an internal hazard only. Substances that emit alpha radiation include uranium, plutonium and radon.

Beta particles: Can penetrate skin and subcutaneous tissue. Clothing will normally protect covered areas. Can cause primary damage to exposed skin and significant burns can occur. Also causes damage if deposited internally. Substances that emit beta radiation include iodine and tritium.

Gamma rays: The most penetrating type of radiation. Can penetrate many centimetres in human tissue. They are the primary cause of acute radiation syndrome.

X-rays: Can penetrate human tissue. Energy level is determined by the voltage to which electrons are accelerated.

Neutrons: Can travel many metres in air and can have a range in tissue to many centimetres according to energy.

Figure 9.13 Ionizing radiation and its risks (Steedman 1994; Eaton 1999)

---

is a potential for contamination, appropriate radiation response protocols should be implemented, and staff should wear protective clothing and respirators where necessary (Wythe 1999).

The principles of treatment are the same whether the casualty is contaminated with radioactive material or toxic chemicals (Dove 1994):

- The physical condition of the casualty takes priority over decontamination procedures.
- The number of staff involved in caring for the patient is kept to a minimum.
- The facilities used are isolated until the patient has been decontaminated.

When dealing with contaminated casualties it is imperative that staff wear the appropriate protective clothing. It is recommended that the following clothing should be worn by staff working in the decontamination area:

- coveralls with theatre greens beneath;
- surgical gloves (two pairs) – tape the inner pair to the coverall sleeves to provide a seal;

- theatre boots – coverall should go over the top of the boot;
- 3M particulate respirator;
- laboratory safety spectacles;
- theatre caps – tuck all hair into cap;
- plastic apron.

The major incident plan relating to radioactive casualties should be initiated in order to reduce the spread of possible contamination throughout the hospital. The on-call Radiation Protection Advisor should be called immediately and requested to attend the Emergency Department. An area should be designated within the Emergency Department to receive and treat contaminated casualties (Steedman 1994). This area should be physically separate from the main area and have its own outside entrance. An alternative method is to use a portable decontamination unit such as the Aireshower by Aireshelta® Limited, as this avoids major disruption to the Emergency Department (see Figure 9.14). Whichever method is utilized, the area must be equipped to deal with resuscitation and emergency procedures. If using an existing area within the Emergency Department ensure that it is closed and sealed to everybody except nominated staff who should be dressed in the appropriate personal protection clothing. The floor of the room must be covered with plastic sheeting that should be taped down to minimize potential contamination, and all non-essential items removed from the room. Radioactive warning signs need to be placed on all doorways and the immediate area cordoned off. The room is divided into a dirty side and a clean side.

Upon receipt of radioactive casualties, the first priority is the treatment of life-threatening injuries. Once the patient has been stabilized then the second priority is the assessment of the extent and magnitude of contamination, and decontamination as necessary (NHSE 1998). The on-call medical physicist, using a mobile contamination monitor, carries out assessment of contamination. It is the responsibility of the medical physicist or nominated person to record details of all contamination found, the relevant levels and various sites involved. Also, they should record details of all personnel in contact with the contaminated area.

The treatment of a contaminated casualty follows similar principles to that of "barrier nursing". The aim of decontamination is to remove radioactive material from the patient's body and to minimize absorption into the body through the mouth, eyes, nose or open wounds (Steedman 1994). Most radioactive material can be removed by thorough washing with soap and running water. All clothing removed from contaminated patients should be bagged, marked "radioactive", secured and labelled with the patient's name. The rules of priority for external decontamination are shown in Figure 9.15. More detailed information on decontamination procedures is outside the scope of this book but is covered in *Planning for major incidents: the NHS guidance* (NHSE 1998). When dealing with internally contaminated casualties it is imperative that the laboratory samples detailed in Figure 9.16 are collected.

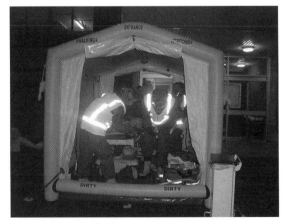

Figure 9.14 Portable decontamination unit

- Remove clothing
- Cover uncontaminated wounds
- Decontaminate in the following order:
  - contaminated wounds
  - nose, eyes, mouth
  - near nose, eyes, mouth
  - near uncontaminated wounds
  - "hot spots" on skin
  - other areas of skin
- Finally, contaminated wounds can be debrided if necessary

Figure 9.15 Rules of priority for external decontamination (Steedman 1994)

A. **Blood** – approximately 20–30 ml for the following analyses:
1 Full blood count
2 Cytogenetic analysis (24 h after exposure)
3 Biochemical analysis (serum amylase)
4 Analysis for radionuclide content
B. **High nasal (bilateral) throat swabs:**
Dry swabs stored in labelled holders without transport medium. They should be taken as early as possible and the time recorded. They will need to be sent to a laboratory specializing in the measurement of radionuclides.
C. **Urine:**
1 Routine analysis
2 Biochemical (creatinurea)
3 Analysis for radionuclide content
D. **Stools (for estimation of radionuclide contents):**
Only those patients with combined injuries and/or a severe prodomal syndrome will require treatment in the reception area.

Figure 9.16 Important laboratory samples to be taken from radiation casualties (NHSE 1998)

INCIDENTS INVOLVING CHEMICALS

There are more than 11 million chemical substances known to man, of which some 60,000 to 70,000 are in regular use (United Nations Environment Programme 1992). With the constant threat of accidental releases of hazardous materials and the potential use of chemical weapons by terrorists, Emergency Departments must be prepared to handle victims who may be contaminated with chemical substances (Olson and Tharrat 1999). Indeed, Steedman (1994) observed that there are at least 30 countries worldwide who have stockpiles of chemical weapons. More worrying is the increasing threat of bio-terrorism, examples of which are the Tokyo sarin gas attack on 20th March 1995 which killed 12 people and injured over 5500, and incidents such as the mercury poisoning of Israeli citrus in 1978, the Tylenol-cyanide poisoning of 1982 and the salmonella poisonings by the Rajneesh cult in Oregon in 1984 (National Research Council 1999).

The need for Emergency Department readiness to deal with chemical incidents is highlighted by Murray (2000). She commented on a report by the Chemical Incident Response Service in 1998 that showed nine health care facilities had to be closed, in part or entirely, as a result of chemical incidents. Various papers (Baxter 1991; Rodgers 1998) have raised concerns about the ability of UK health services to cope with incidents involving hazardous chemicals and more specifically, Horby et al (2000) identified serious deficiencies in English Emergency Departments'

ability to respond to chemical incidents. Lessons learnt from the Sarin gas attack in Tokyo in 1995 highlight the potentially devastating effect that contaminated casualties can have on Emergency Department staff with 13 of the 15 doctors treating casualties being adversely affected by symptoms (Nozaki et al 1995).

A chemical incident is defined as,

"An unforeseen event, involving non-radioactive substances, that results in potential toxic risk to public health, or leads to the exposure of two or more individuals and results in illness or potential illness, or two or more individuals suffering from a similar illness that might be attributable to such an event" (Fisher et al 1999).

One of the major problems in planning for chemical incidents is the lack of comprehensive sources of information on their frequency and nature (Palmer et al 2000). A prospective study by Maclean (1981) identified an average of three chemical incidents and two casualties per day in the UK. Bowen (1998) identified 369 separate chemical incidents between the years 1980 and 1997, over 50% of which occurred in the USA and the UK. The varying types of chemical incident and their frequency as determined by Bowen (1998) are shown in Tables 9.2 and 9.3. Murray (2000) argues that the NHS guidance, *Planning for major incidents* (NHSE 1998) places an onus upon Emergency Departments to carry out a full risk assessment of chemical hazards within their geographical boundaries.

Major disasters and major incidents

Table 9.2 Type of chemical incident – fixed facility (%)	
Chemical plant	72
Storage	11
Commercial premises	7
Farms	5
Water treatment works	3
Waste disposal sites	2

Table 9.3 Type of chemical incident – transport related (%)	
Rail	41
Highway	32
Sea	18
Pipeline	9

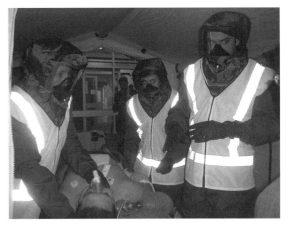

Figure 9.17 Chemical protective suits

Chemical disasters are unique in that contaminated casualties pose the problem of cross-contamination of the chemical to emergency services and Emergency Department personnel (Totenhofer and Kierce 1999). Therefore, whenever dealing with chemical incidents, and the resultant casualties, it is imperative that emergency nursing staff think safety first. All Emergency Departments should possess chemical protective suits and respirators for the protection of nursing and medical staff involved in decontamination procedures (NHSE 1998). The Ambulance Service Association Chemical Incident Procedures Working Group (1998) has produced useful guidance on suitable personal chemical protective equipment. The TST-Sweden chemical protection suit is commonly used by many emergency services and is shown in Figure 9.17. Coates et al (1999) concluded that it was feasible to perform life-saving procedures whilst wearing such a suit after a study in the Royal Preston Hospital.

Chemical injury depends on the concentration or strength of the agent, the amount involved and the manner and duration of contact (Totenhofer and Kierce 1999). Chemical exposure may occur via three major routes; by oral ingestion, by inhalation, and by absorption following skin contact (Timbrell 1999). Rapid decontamination and first aid are essential as chemical action can be progressive and continues until any active chemicals are inactivated (Degg 1997). The most effective decontamination is that done within the first few minutes after exposure; it can mean the

difference between minimal or severe injury for the patient or even life or death (MRICD 1995). Ideally, the decontamination of casualties should take place as close to the incident scene as possible (NHSE 1998). In most circumstances it is the agreed responsibility of the Fire and Rescue Service to decontaminate contaminated casualties at the scene of the incident (Eaton 2000). However, Saunders and Ward (2000) suggest that Fire Service decontamination units are designed for fire fighters in full protective gear and are inappropriate for unprotected casualties. Regardless of pre-hospital decontamination in a disaster, the Emergency Department would expect to receive a number of "walk in" contaminated casualties (Totenhofer and Kierce 1999).

Chemical agents may cause multi-system effects and it is therefore imperative to ascertain the type of chemical involved in a chemical incident as soon as possible. The Control of Industrial Major Accident Hazard Regulations 1984 mean that information should be readily and speedily available for an incident occurring at a hazardous industrial site from the onsite safety plan. For incidents involving the transportation of hazardous chemicals, identification can be made either by the transport emergency (TREM) cards, which are held in the drivers cab, or by the HAZCHEM codes displayed on the back and sides of the vehicle.

Further detailed information about toxic chemicals and their treatments can be obtained from the National Poisons Information Service (see Figure 9.18), through Toxbase, which is a computerized information guide

Mike Hayward

London	0207 6359191
Cardiff	01222 709901
Belfast	01232 240503
Edinburgh	0131 5362300

Figure 9.18 Telephone numbers of National Poisons Information Service

containing information about 8000 products, or through CHEMDATA, the fire service's fax link to the national chemical advisory service.

The principles of decontamination are similar to when dealing with radioactive casualties. Remember think safety first, always approach casualties from upwind and uphill if possible. The casualty should be moved to a well-ventilated and protected area. If decontamination is to be carried out at the Emergency Department then it should be carried out in a portable decontamination unit outside the department, or inside a specially designed decontamination room within the department.

Decontamination is accomplished by the removal of the agent by physical means or by chemical neutralization or detoxification (MRICD 1995). Running water, or more preferably, low-pressure showers should be used for most decontaminations, but care must be exercised not to cause excessive splashing of the chemical contaminant. Thorough information about the type of contamination present must be established prior to using water decontamination as certain chemicals react with water. If a water volatile chemical is involved then a dry decontamination procedure must be used. Again, as with radioactive contamination, the patient's clothes must be sealed in a plastic bag and clearly labelled as a hazard.

Although chemical incidents are rare, evidence presented earlier demonstrates that they do occur, and that most Emergency Departments are inadequately prepared or trained to deal with them (Rodgers 1998; Totenhofer and Kierce 1999). There is clearly a need for emergency nurses to take the initiative and adequately prepare for dealing with chemically contaminated casualties if they are not themselves to become secondary casualties (Rodgers 1998). Emergency Departments must have written and easily implemented procedures as part of their disaster policy, coupled with the appropriate equipment and training (Totenhofer and Kierce 1999). Therefore, the

role of education and training for all types of major incident or disaster cannot be overemphasized.

PLANNING, TRAINING AND EDUCATION

Guidance for emergency planning in the NHS for England has been regularly supplied and updated for many years (DoH 1989; NHSME 1990; NHSE 1996; 1998). Detailed examination of these documents reveals a lack of clear advice and instruction on assessing the local hazards and risks. Indeed, the current NHS guidance, *Planning for major incidents* devotes only one page to this important area of planning. Unfortunately, as with much NHS guidance, it is aimed at regional strategists and planners rather than offering "coal face" workers such emergency nurses practical help and advice. Whilst Regional Health Authorities often have risk profiles of many potential disaster hazards such as oil refineries, football grounds and chemical plants, this data is not commonly located in many Emergency Departments for access by nursing staff.

Insufficient training and preparation have repeatedly been cited as problems in the preparation for major incidents in the UK (Carley and Mackway-Jones 1996; Nancekievill 1992). This is no longer acceptable and is spelt out by the NHSE (1998, p. 20) who state that, "High standards will be expected from: front line responders – for example, the ambulance service and mobile medical teams and receiving hospitals". Earlier guidance from the NHSE (1996) had also reinforced that listed hospitals and ambulance services in England and Wales have a legal responsibility to make a plan, train staff, and to exercise their plan.

Savage (1979) highlights that many hospital major incident plans have failed in the past because the plans were too dependent on one or two named individuals. Although most hospital major incident plans have moved away from named individuals in specific roles to the concept of staff action cards, it is still individuals that can spell disaster for major incident training and preparation. All too often the NHSE (1998) document *Planning for major incidents* is locked away in Chief Executives or Emergency Department Consultants' offices, the true details of major incident plans are often a complete mystery to most staff and there is little in-house training provided by many nominated Emergency Planning Liaison Officers. There are notable exceptions to this in various Emergency Departments in the UK; Redmond (1989), and King and James (2000) cite examples of multi-disciplinary training and regular practice drills.

As stated earlier in this chapter, a majority of hospital staff responding to a major incident, whether as a member of MMT or as part of a receiving hospital, will have no previous experience of such an event. Therefore, the lack of previous experience necessitates good planning and rehearsal of major incident roles (Carley and Mackway-Jones 1997a, b).

TRAINING AND EDUCATIONAL RECOMMENDATIONS

The following recommendations are made as a suggested guide for training and effective staff preparedness in the Emergency Department for major incidents:

- The senior emergency nurse and at least two other senior emergency nurses to have attended a MIMMS course.
- A senior emergency nurse to be the nominated major incident and disaster planning lead.
- Establish links with the regional Health Emergency Planning Advisor (HEPA).
- The formation of a multi-disciplinary major incident training team (to include all grades of nursing staff).
- Regular in-house training and study days (training to include possible types of disaster scenario, roles of staff in major incident, awareness of the NHS guidance, scene command, role of MMTs, familiarization of equipment).
- Detailed risk assessment of all potential hazards and risks in catchment area of hospital (to include chemical plants, oil refineries, high rise flats, railway lines, motorways, nightclubs, large sporting venues, military establishments, nuclear installations, ports and docks, airports, armament depots and fuel depots).
- All staff to be given a copy of the Emergency Department major incident plan on induction.
- MMT equipment and drugs to be checked monthly and stored in an easily accessible manner.

- Regular liaison with other pre-hospital emergency providers such as the fire service, police and ambulance service to enhance understanding of roles and nurture more efficient cross service working.
- Nomination of potential staff for the MMT role at the beginning of each shift as a matter of routine.
- All staff should have easy access to the document, *Planning for major incidents – The NHS guidance* (NHSE 1998).
- The Emergency Department major incident plan should be tested at least twice per year.

References

Advanced Life Support Group (1995) *Major incident medical management and support – the practical approach.* London: BMJ Publishing group.

Ambulance Service Association Chemical Incident Procedures Working Group (1998) *Guidance on chemical incidents.* ASA.

Baxter PJ (1991) Major chemical disasters. Britain's health services are poorly prepared. *Br Med J* 302: 61–62.

Bliss A (1984) Major disaster planning. *Br Med J* 288: 1433–1434.

Bowen HJ (1998) *A public health management model for acute chemical incidents in Wales.* Ph.D. dissertation, Open University.

British Broadcasting Corporation (BBC) (2001) New anthrax victim gravely ill. Accessed on 16th May at: http://news.bbc.co.uk/hi/english/world/americas/newsid_1612000/1612395.stm.

British Energy (undated) Available from: http://www.british-energy.com/media/mn_factfiles_transport.html accessed 12th Mar. 2001.

Carley SD, Mackway-Jones K (1996) Are British hospitals ready for the next major incident? Analysis of hospital major incident plans. *Br Med J* 313: 1242–1243.

Carley SD, Mackway-Jones K (1997a) The casualty profile from the Manchester bombing 1996: a proposal for the construction and dissemination of casualty profiles from major incidents. *J Accid Emergen Med* 14: 76–80.

Carley SD, Mackway-Jones K (1997b) The preparation for the pre-hospital surgical and non-surgical response to major incidents in the United Kingdom. *Pre-Hosp Immed Care* 1: 68–70.

Carley S, Mackway-Jones K, Donnan S (1998) Major incidents in Britain over the past 28 years: the case for centralised reporting of major incidents. *J Epidemiol Commun Health* 52: 392–398.

Clarke RH (1987) Dose distributions in Western Europe following Chernobyl. In: Jones RR, Southwood R, eds. *Radiation and health.* Chichester: John Wiley and Sons.

Clifton NJ (1994) The M1 plane crash – managing the hospital response. In: Wallace WA, Rowles JM, Colton CL, eds. *Management of disasters and their aftermath.* London: BMJ Publishing Group.

Coates MJ, Ayman SJ, James MR (1999) Chemical protective clothing; a study into the ability of staff to perform lifesaving procedures. *J Accid Emergen Med* 17: 115–118.

Cooke MW (1992) Arrangements for on scene medical care at major incidents. *Br Med J* 305: 748.

Crouch R, Marrow J (1996) Towards a UK triage scale. *Emergen Nurs* 4(3): 4–5.

Davis J, Stewart L (2000) Air flight disaster, post traumatic stress, and post ventive rescue and response: the aftermath of the San Diago PSA 182 plane crash recovery operation, 20 years on. *Accid Emergen Nurs* 8: 13–19.

Degg S (1997) *Chemical burns, toxic chemical incidents: a symposium*. Victoria: Australia Disaster College.

Department of Health (1989) *Health services development. Emergency planning in the NHS. Health services arrangements for dealing with accidents involving radioactivity*. HC(89)8/HN(FP)(89)8, London: HMSO.

Department of Health and Social Services (Public Safety Unit) (2000) *Integrated emergency management for health and personal social services in Northern Ireland*. PSU1/2000.

Dove AF (1994) Dealing with chemical and radioactive decontamination in major disasters. In: Wallace WA, Rowles JM, Colton CL, eds. *Management of disasters and their aftermath*. London: BMJ Publishing Group.

Eaton CJ (1999) *Essentials of immediate medical care*. Edinburgh: Churchill Livingstone.

Fennell QC, D (1988) *Investigation into the King's cross underground fire*. London: HMSO (CM499).

Fisher J, Morgan-Jones D, Murray V, Davies G (1999) *Chemical incident management for accident and emergency clinicians*. London: HMSO.

Fletcher V (1986) When the music stopped. *Nurs Times* April 30: 30–32.

Fong F, Schrader DC (1996) Radiation disasters and emergency department preparedness. *Disast Med* 14(2): 349–370.

Fry FA (1987) Doses from environmental radioactivity. In: Jones RR, Southwood R, eds. *Radiation and health*. Chichester: John Wiley and Sons.

Geologyshop.co.uk. (undated) Available from: http://www.geologyshop.co.uk/ukequakes.htm accessed 12th Mar. 2001.

Graham CA, Hearns ST (1999) Major incidents: training for on site medical personnel. *J Accid Emergen Med* 16: 336–338.

Health and Safety Executive (1974) *Health and safety at work act*. London: HSE.

Hidden QC, A (1989) *Investigation into the Clapham junction railway accident*. London: HMSO (CM820).

Hines K (1997) The medical management of major incidents – past, present and future. *J Br Assoc Immed Care* 20: 1–6.

Hinks M (1993) We went to see Liverpool get to Wembley: the experience of a Hillsborough Survivor. In: Newburn T, ed. *Working with disaster – social welfare interventions during and after tragedy*. Harlow: Longman Group UK.

Hodgetts T, Miles S (2000) Major incidents. In: Driscoll P, Skinner D, Earlam R, eds. *ABC of major trauma* 3rd ed. London: BMJ Books.

Horby P, Murray V, Cummins A, Mackway-Jones K, Euripidou R (2000) The capability of accident and emergency departments to safely decontaminate victims of chemical incidents. *J Accid Emergen Med* 17: 344–347.

International Federation of Red Cross and Red Crescent Societies (2000) *World disasters report. Focus on public health*. Geneva: International Federation of Red Cross and Red Crescent Societies.

Kilner T (1996) Equipping the pre-hospital care team. *Emergen Nurs* 3(4): 16–19.

Kilner T (2000) Pre-hospital care. In: Dolan B, Holt L, eds. *Accident and emergency – theory into practice*. Edinburgh: Bailliere Tindall.

Lloyd D (1991) Cannon street rail crash: a report by the director of operations. London Ambulance Service, unpublished. Cited in: New B (1992). *Too many cooks? The response of the health-related services to major incidents in London*. Research Report 15. London: Kings Fund Institute.

Lumley JSP (1998) Disater mitigation. In: Greaves I, Ryan JM, Porter KM, eds. *Trauma*. London: Edward Arnold.

McGregor P, Driscoll P, Sammy I et al (1997) Are UK mobile medical teams safe? *Pre-Hosp Immed Care* 1: 183–188.

Mackway-Jones K, ed. (1996) *Emergency triage: Manchester Triage Group*. London: BMJ.

Maclean AD (1981) Chemical incidents handled by the United Kingdom public fire service in 1980. *J Hazard Mater* 5: 3–40.

Marriott PB (1991) *Report of the Chief Inspector of Marine Accidents into the collision between the passenger launch Marchioness and MV Bowbelle*. London: The Department of Transport, HMSO.

Medical Research Institute of Chemical Defence (1995) *Medical management of chemical casualties handbook* 2nd ed. Maryland: US Army.

Moakes S, Kilner T (2001) Nurses' understanding of their role as part of a mobile medical and nursing team during a major incident. *Pre-Hosp Immed Care* 5(1): 34–37.

Murray V (2000) Chemical incidents. In: Driscoll P, Skinner D, Earlam R, eds. *ABC of major trauma* 3rd ed. London: BMJ Books.

Nancekievill DG (1992) On site medical services at major incidents. *Br Med J* 305: 721–727.

National Research Council – Institute of Medicine (1999) *Chemical and biological terrorism: research and development to improve civilian medical response*. Washington, DC: National Academy Press, p. 15.

New B (1992) *Too many cooks? The response of the health-related services to major incidents in London*. Research Report 15. London: Kings Fund Institute.

NHS Directorate for the National Assembly for Wales (1999) *Planning for major incidents: the NHS guidance*. WHC(99)155, Cardiff, NHS Directorate for the National Assembly for Wales.

NHSE (1996) Emergency planning in the NHS: *health services arrangements for dealing with major incidents* Vol. 1. London: Emergency planning co-ordination unit, NHS Executive.

NHSE (1998) *Planning for major incidents – the NHS guidance*. London: NHS Executive.

NHSME (1990) *Emergency planning in the NHS: health services arrangements for dealing with major incidents*. London: NHS Management Executive, HC 90(25).

NHS in Scotland (1998) *Manual of guidance: responding to emergencies*. Edinburgh: The Scottish Office.

Mike Hayward

Norton C (1998) Safety considerations for nursing staff on a mobile medical/nursing team. *A&E Focus* 9: 3–5.

Nozaki H, Hori S, Shinozawa YFS et al (1995) Secondary exposure of medical staff to sarin vapour in the emergency room. *Inten Care Med* 21: 1032–1035.

Olson KR, Tharrat SR (1999) Emergency medical response to hazardous materials incidents. In: Olson KR, Anderson IB, Neal L, Benowitz PD, Clark RF, Kearney TE, Osterich JD, eds. *Poisoning and drug overdose*. Stamford: Appleton and Lange.

Palmer SR, Rees H, Coleman G (2000) Major chemical incidents: bridging the occupational–public health gap. *Occup Med* 50(4): 221–225.

Readers Digest (1991) *Universal dictionary*. London: The Reader's Digest Association Limited, p. 442.

Ricks RC, Fry SA, eds. (1990) *The medical basis for radiation accident preparedness II: clinical experience and follow up since 1979*. New York: Elsevier.

Rodgers J (1998) A chemical gas incident in London. How well prepared are London A&E departments to deal effectively with such an event? *Accid Emergen Nurs* 6: 82–86.

Rutherford WH, de Boer J (1983) The definition and classification of disasters. *Injury* 15: 10–12.

Ryan J, Gavalas M (1998) What goes wrong at a disaster or major incident? *Hosp Med* 59(12): 944–946.

Saunders P, Ward G (2000) Decontamination of chemically contaminated casualties: implications for the health service and a regional strategy. *Pre-Hosp Immed Care* 4: 122–125.

Savage PEA (1979) *Disasters – hospital planning. A manual for doctors, nurses and administrators*. Oxford: Pergamon Press.

Salt P (1989) The mobile medical team. In: Walsh M, ed. *Disasters – current planning and recent experience*. London: Edward Arnold.

Sleet R (1989) Multi-disciplinary teamwork and communication. In: Walsh M, ed. *Disasters – current planning and recent experience*. London: Edward Arnold.

Smith R (1995) Smuggling of plutonium poses major health threat. *Br Med J* 310: 485.

Steedman DJ (1994) *Environmental medical emergencies*. Oxford: Oxford University Press.

The League of Red Cross and Red Crescent Societies (1985) *Guidelines for nurses in disaster preparedness and relief*. Geneva: The League of Red Cross and Red Crescent Societies.

The New Shorter Oxford English Dictionary (1993) Oxford: Clarendon Press, p. 683.

The Times Newspaper (2001, September 12th) America awakes to terrorism by timetable – and the darkest national catastrophe. A tragedy unfolds by Michael Grove. *The Times*, p. 1.

Tierney KJ (1989) The social and community contexts of disaster. In: Gist R, Lubin B, eds. *Psychosocial aspects of disaster*. New York: John Wiley and Sons, pp. 11–12.

Timbrell JA (1999) *Introduction to toxicology*. London: Taylor and Francis.

Torro.co.uk. (undated) Available from: http://www.torro.org.uk/extremes.htm accessed 12th Mar. 2001.

Totenhofer RI, Kierce M (1999) It's a disaster: emergency departments' preparation for a chemical incident or disaster. *Accid Emergen Nurs* 7: 141–147.

United Nations Environment Programme (1992) *Chemical pollution: a global overview*. The international register of potentially toxic chemicals and the global environment monitoring and assessment research centre. Geneva: United Nations.

Wallace AW (1994) It couldn't happen to us. In: Wallace AW, Rowles JM, Colton CL, eds. *Management of disasters and their aftermath*. London: BMA Publishing, p. 1.

Walsh M (1989) *Disasters – current planning and recent experience*. London: Edward Arnold.

Walsh M (1990) *Accident and emergency nursing – a new approach*. Oxford: Butterworth Heinemann.

Whitfield A, Kilner T (2000) Major incident planning. In: Dolan B, Holt L, eds. *Accident and emergency – theory into practice*. Edinburgh: Baillière Tindall.

World Health Organisation (WHO) (1999) *Development of a disaster preparedness tool kit for nursing and midwifery*. Report of a WHO meeting, Coleraine, United Kingdom, 20–21 August 1999. European Health 21, Target 18.

Wythe ET (1999) Specific poisons and drugs: diagnosis and treatment. In: Olson KR, Anderson IB, Neal L, Benowitz PD, Clark RF, Kearney TE, Osterich JD, eds. *Poisoning and drug overdose*. Stamford: Appleton and Lange.

Major disasters and major incidents

Index